THE VISUAL HANDBOOK

THE COMPLETE GUIDE TO SEEING MORE CLEARLY

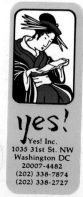

yes!

Yes! Inc.
1035 31st St. NW
Washington DC
20007-4482
(202) 338-7874
(202) 338-2727

N
2-91

By the same author
FINDING EACH OTHER

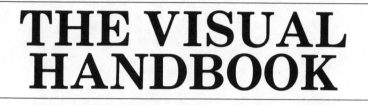

THE VISUAL HANDBOOK

THE COMPLETE GUIDE TO SEEING MORE CLEARLY

John Selby

Element Books

Printed and bound in Great Britain
by Billings, Hylton Road, Worcester

Designed by Jenny Liddle

Cover illustration: Chinese Whispers by Diane Fisher

British Library Cataloguing in Publication Data
Selby, John
The visual handbook: the complete guide
to seeing more clearly.
1. Vision disorders – Treatment
2. Selfcare, Health
I. Title   II. Das Gesundheitsbuch fur
die Augen. *English*
617.7'068   RE61

ISBN 1-85230-018-3

CONTENTS

PROLOGUE viii

INTRODUCTION x

PART ONE **VISUAL HEALTH AND ENHANCED PERFORMANCE**

1. THE ART OF SEEING 3

2. EXPANDING OUR PERCEPTION.................................24

3. VISUALIZATION: THE EYES AND THE MIND..........32

4. VISUAL HEALTH AND PHYSICAL HEALTH.............38

5. VISUAL HEALTH AND EMOTIONAL HEALTH.........50

6. RELAXATION 57

7. LIGHT, LIGHTING, AND EYE-STRAIN REDUCTION 62

8. COMMON VISUAL DIFFICULTIES...........................67

9. ENHANCING THE PLEASURE OF SEEING.................73

10. REVIEW AND PROGRAMMES 77

PART TWO **VISUAL TREATMENT AND RECOVERY PROGRAMME**

INTRODUCTION WHEN PROBLEMS APPEAR 93

11. NEAR-SIGHTEDNESS (Myopia).........................94

12. FAR-SIGHTEDNESS (Hyperopia and Presbyopia) 127

13. CATARACTS ('Old Age Blindness')................................140

14. THE GLAUCOMAS (Inner Eye Pressure).......................150

15. CROSS-EYES AND WANDERING EYES (Strabismus) 160

16. EYE ALLERGIES (Conjunctivitis) 169
17. THE RETINA: MIRACLES AND TRAGEDIES............176
18. FINAL WORDS...187
   BIBLIOGRAPHY 191

Author Profile

John Selby, born in California in 1945, is a psychologist specializing in the emotional and environmental causes of physical disorders. Having recovered his own clear eyesight after a decade of short-sightedness and astigmatism, one of his primary research and therapy focuses has been the treatment of visual disorders.

Selby obtained his undergraduate degree in developmental psychology from Princeton University in 1968, and then did graduate work at the University of California at Berkeley (Master's degree) before studying comparative healing traditions at the San Francisco Theological Seminary and the Graduate Theological Union. He finished his professional studies at the Radix Institute in Ojai, California.

The author's professional posts have included research at the New Jersey Neuro-psychiatric Institute, the Bureau of Research in Neurology and Psychiatry, and the American Institute for Mental Health. A past director of the American Institute for Visual Health, Selby has also developed health and vision programmes for the American Airline Pilots' Association, Aetna Life Insurance, IBM, and Apple Computers.

Concurrent with research and private practice (the San Luis Obispo Holistic Health Center; the Reid Vision Center) Selby has written numerous books during the last fifteen years, including *The Holistic Handbook of Therapeutic Massage* (Kent Books, 1970); *Visionetics* (with Lisette Scholl, Doubleday/Dolphin, 1977); a health-oriented novel, *Powerpoint* (Warner Books 1981); and the *See Clearly Book* (Vision Press, 1982). His most recent books are *Responsive Breathing* (Sphinx Verlag in Basel, 1984) and *Visual Health and Recovery* (Scherz Verlag in Bern, 1985), *Finding Each Other* (Element Books, 1987), and *The Heart of Immune-System Activation* (Droemer/Knaur, 1987).

PROLOGUE

My intention in writing this present book, my fourth on vision, has been to offer a broad, comprehensive view of how our eyes function, how they sometimes misfunction, and how we can act to regain optimum visual health and vitality.

While giving adequate attention to the seven most common visual disorders in our culture, I have also saved space for a more positive exploration of how all of us, regardless of our visual condition, can actively improve our visual potential, and regain the pleasure and spontaneity of seeing which we all knew during our early years of life.

Finally, I have presented a simple explanation of the treatments and procedures you can expect when you turn to the medical community for help with a visual problem, and also a basic introduction to the personal healing techniques which you can use yourself to encourage your healing process.

Each of you, of course, has a particular reason for picking up this book. Some of you have definite eye problems which you want to understand better, in which case you will probably want practical advice on which treatments might best serve you. Some of you have no vision problems as such, but would like to improve your general perception habits and expand your pleasure in seeing. Finally, some of you simply want to know how your eyes work, and how you can act on your own to preserve your eyesight in optimum health throughout your lives.

Rather than simply updating the traditional discussions on how eyes work and how visual diseases sometimes develop, I have tried to make this book much more enjoyable. Especially, I have focused considerable attention on the inner aspects of seeing, to the relationship between your emotions, your mental states, and your seeing habits.

With every passing hour, more and more doctors and scientists agree that our emotional habits, our mental states, and our behaviour patterns influence our health and vitality in a direct and powerful manner. New programmes have been developed which give guidance in self-help at these levels, so that inner states can encourage healing, rather than getting in its way.

Also, you will find in this book a number of practical programmes which link your conscious desire for clear vision with your biochemical functioning. These are still at the experimental stage, but they point towards major breakthroughs in physical health and are completely safe for you to use on your own.

It should be stated at the outset, however, that the more advanced recovery programmes presented here are not meant to replace traditional medical treatment. Rather it is the integration of medical with psychological treatments which affords optimum healing potential.

Naturally, a book such as this does not arise from the work and research of a single individual, and I would like to express my deep appreciation to the wide range of professionals and scientists who have added their insights and technical understanding to the present discussion. I would also like to thank at this point the hundreds of clients who have explored various healing techniques with my colleagues and myself, and who have been pioneers in their own right in the field of visual health and recovery.

I would also like to thank the growing number of doctors throughout the country who are expanding their concepts of treatment to include the psychological factor in healing. This book is not intended to be opposed to the traditional medical community, and I certainly hope that the programmes offered here are welcomed as supplementary to the existing medical treatments. I also hope that my explanations of the various visual complications help doctor and patient to communicate more clearly and to work together towards the common goal of recovery.

Especially, I hope that each page of this book is enjoyable for you to read, informative, and insightful as well. Vision is an infinite experience, and any discussion of eyesight needs to include the various depths of visual experience which are possible. Thus, along with quite medical discussions, you will also find in this book occasional visual meditations, which offer you a pathway into new experiences of who you are, and how vision reflects deeper levels of consciousness.

Finally, before we move on to the actual exploration of your eyesight, I would like to express my deep thanks to my son, Sean, who is sleeping patiently through the clatter of my typing. May his generation have an easier time of healing and seeing clearly than past generations. And may the eyesight of the new generations be such that they can see clearly to the heart of things, and act accordingly!

John Selby

INTRODUCTION

We receive over 70 per cent of our sensory experiences through our eyes. Most of our physical movements, our emotional responses, our mental performance, and even our deeper spiritual insights, are intimately linked with the successful functioning of our visual system. Because of this vital dependency on eyesight, it is natural that we want to preserve our vision in optimum condition.

Almost all of us are born with healthy eyesight. Aside from infrequent genetic complications, we enter this world with the inherent ability and desire to see clearly.

However, as we proceed through our lives, many of us begin to develop visual complications which interfere both with our ability to see clearly, and also our enjoyment in seeing. Such complications emerge not only from genetic factors, but also from our perception habits developed as children, environmental conditions which generate stress, and our emotional atmosphere, which creates powerful subconscious reverberations throughout our bodies.

Even if we can see clearly in optometric tests, a large number of us have ingrained visual habits which interfere with optimal perception, generating eye-strain and headache, reducing our visual processing skills, and interfering with our enjoyment of seeing the world around us.

Our ability to see clearly is a variable which we can actively enhance, regardless of our visual condition at the time. Whether we are 10 years old or 80, we can still actively help our eyesight to remain vital, healthy, and stimulating. The purpose of this book is to offer you a practical, comprehensive guide for gaining and maintaining such optimum visual health, efficiency, and enjoyment.

Although we will consider in depth the optometric, surgical, and pharmacological treatments for various vision disorders, the bias of this book is in favour of your doing whatever is possible to help yourself first, before turning to medical intervention. And even while being treated medically, you can continue to augment this treatment with your own conscious efforts.

When you were very young, your eyes were in a state of relative bliss.

They were completely free to look wherever they wanted to, to explore the visual world without control and inhibitions. A natural spontaneity existed visually, a quality which gave basic vitality and health to the eyes. Seeing was a pleasure, the eyes remained relaxed, active, full of curiosity and joy.

But subsequent years brought about quite different developments in your experience of seeing. Especially when you went off to school, your eyes quickly became prisoners, slaves forced to perform difficult, tiring, uninteresting jobs for hours on end, with the threat of punishment hanging overhead if the repetitive tasks were not performed.

The loss of spontaneity which occurs visually when children are sent to school has been considered one of the necessary side effects of our advanced civilization. Without forcing the eyes to work as slaves hour after hour, our present educational and economic system might not function at all. So we continue to treat our eyes very badly, forcing them to perform against their natural tendencies, passing on this habitual pattern generation after generation.

It now appears more and more probable that a large number of our visual problems are at least a partial result of this forced constriction in childhood. The eye problems might manifest themselves early, as in childhood myopia, of later, in various forms of visual constriction and malfunctioning. But when we look for causes in visual disfunctioning, tension, stress, anxiety, and other habitual inhibitions seem to be primary suspects.

We need to gain a fuller understanding of both the genetic, environmental, and also emotional factors which influence our health, and our visual health in particular. We need to give our eyes more freedom, to break out of habitual tension patterns in seeing, and to bring back the sense of spontaneity which our eyes enjoyed when we were very young.

Traditionally, exercises for the eyes have been anything but spontaneous pleasures. They have been difficult, boring, anxiety-provoking, and in general the opposite of what the eyes are yearning for.

This present series of exercises and vision programmes is designed to be enjoyable, satisfying, and insightful. The aim is to free the eyes, not to further condition them. If you approach the exercises and healing sessions in the traditional way, forcing your eyes to do something for their own good, you will negate the possible benefits. Instead, you should take a deep breath, give yourself permission to have a good time, and then delve into the experiences which might come forth as you are exploring your visual potential.

Each of us has a particular unique set of perceptual habits which reflect our deeper personalities. The way in which we look at the world is an expression of our basic view of the world. Therefore, as you use the exercises in this book to expand your perceptual habits, you are actually expanding your personality, your range of consciousness, as well.

This is perhaps the most exciting aspect of this form of growth – a simple vision exercise, such as presented in Chapter 1, can suddenly generate a resonating expansion of the entire personality. In fact, the exercises presented in this book are part of a personality-growth programme directly aimed at the rapid expansion of personality and consciousness. So as you help your eyes, you help yourself in general.

It is this intimate interplay between your eyes, and the rest of your being, which underlies the entire discussion of this book. If your eyes were simply isolated organs, not influenced by your thoughts, your feelings, and your whole-body movements, vision would in fact be a very simple affair. But the reality is quite the opposite. Every thought you think, every emotion that rushes through your body, and every movement which you make or don't make brings about a response in your eyes.

We are now going to turn to the first aspect of vision, to the actual experience you are having at this very moment as you read this book. In fact, with every page you read, the focus will naturally return to your own eyes, to your own experience of seeing in the present moment.

How do your eyes feel?

PART ONE
Visual Health and Enhanced Performance

1 · THE ART OF SEEING

To begin our exploration of seeing, we should take a first look at how your own eyes are functioning, right now. By observing your present reading habits, you can gain quite a remarkable insight into your deeper visual world, regardless of your visual condition.

For instance, your eyes are busy right now, moving along these lines of print, taking in the visual information which you need to understand the meaning of this paragraph. The first question we need to consider is whether your eyes are enjoying this reading task, or if they feel like slaves who are being forced to work against their will.

As already mentioned, we tend to treat our eyes very badly, to force them to work, rather than allowing them to take in the world around them spontaneously. If this is true in your case, perhaps it would be best to begin this exploration of your eyesight by making a friendly gesture towards your eyes.

See what happens if you give your eyes permission, right now, to close if they want to, or to look somewhere beyond this page. Take a deep breath, and see how your eyes are in fact feeling right now. And allow them to return to the next paragraph only when they choose to. After all, if your eyes don't want to read this book, how will this book help your eyes? So just explore what happens when you give your eyes more freedom.

Hopefully, as you read through this book, your eyes will regain their lost sense of freedom, and will perform the task of reading with less tension. Just this simple shift in functioning can make a considerable difference in the vitality of your visual system.

BREATHING

Another primary factor we can introduce right at the beginning, to give your eyes a major boost towards optimum health and functioning, is the factor of breathing. As you are reading this paragraph, are you aware of your breathing? Many of us hold our breath or breathe in tight, shallow breaths when we read. This is because reading was associated with tensions and anxieties when we were learning to read, and we still carry these habits with us unconsciously throughout our lives if we don't consciously change them.

So notice as you are reading right now how you are breathing. Is your breathing smooth and deep, or is it irregular, shallow, and high in the chest? Just observe the air coming in and out your nose right now, and feel the movements in your chest and abdomen.

As soon as you become aware of your breathing, it often changes for the better, becoming deeper, more relaxed, and smoother. This shift in the breathing directly affects your overall functioning. If your breathing is tense, so is your body in general. and this includes your eye muscles as well!

Now, while remaining aware of your breathing, also become aware of the movement of your eyes as you read this paragraph. Allow your breathing to be smooth and relaxed, and your eye movements to be relaxed also, so that the act of reading doesn't generate tension. Give your eyes freedom to move along the lines in whatever ways they want to right now. And notice how your breathing responds to different speeds of reading.

The ability to be aware of your eyes seems very simple. But in fact, most people with vision problems have considerable difficulty in focusing on the presence of their eyes, the actual physical presence of the two organs in the head. There are many emotional reasons for this, which we will explain later. For now, it is enough to begin to bring your focus to your eyes gently, through remaining aware of your breathing also.

A primary suggestion at this point is that you don't start judging your performance on any of these exercises. Instead, it is to your advantage simply to observe how you actually do function in the present, and accept this current level. In this state of acceptance, you can then do the exercises and allow your eyes to grow and recover step by step.

You will notice that the basic exercise of being aware of your breathing and your eyes while you read generates an expansion in your consciousness which can be quite beneficial. See if, throughout this book, you can remember to include this awareness while you are reading, and notice how your eyes feel as a result.

AWARENESS OF TIME

Along with breathing and seeing, we can introduce another basic character in this discussion – your perception of the flow of time. Are you hurrying right now as you read this page? Is there some unseen pressure pushing you to read rapidly, to take in the words almost so fast that their impact can't really sink in and affect you?

There are two different ways of reading. With the most popular one these days, you are supposed to read just as fast as you possibly can, picking up the basic meaning of the paragraph, without bothering with individual words. In this way, you can process the maximum amount of information possible.

But there is another way of reading, which should prove more worthwhile for you in reading this book. Intentionally, I am writing words on this page which can have an emotional impact on you if you really explore the suggestions. You are reading this book for the same reason, I suspect. You want to gain something from the experience of reading these pages.

So we should work together, rather than allowing old reading habits to interfere with our communication. To read as rapidly as possible reduces the emotional and intuitive impact that words can have as you read them. So what happens if you slow down your reading rate right now, and allow your reflection on your own eyesight to have some time and space to mature, even while you are reading?

Vision, after all, requires both space and time, in order to function. Seeing is an interaction of these two aspects of life. If we distort or negate one of these aspects, then our experience of seeing is seriously impaired. And quite often, I have found with a majority of clients over the years, tensions involved in the pressures of time are the same tensions which are negatively influencing the health of our eyes.

For this reason, I am starting this book with this rather unusual topic of attention – your breathing, the speed at which you are reading these words, and the extent to which you allow yourself time to reflect on what you are reading, as you read the words.

Let's do another experiment with your eyes. After reading this paragraph, I would like you to pause for four breath cycles and close your eyes. Once they are closed. see if they really want to open again and continue looking out at the world, or if they actually would prefer to remain closed. Begin to give your eyes some freedom, to do what they want to do, and see how well-integrated your eyes are with your general interests and desires. Go ahead and close your eyes right now, and see what experiences come to you, what insights you might gain when you observe your eyes functioning, without judging them, See you in four breaths!

Now as you read these next words, notice if your eyes are moving effortlessly across the page, at a speed which seems to happen without any force. Continue reading while you give your eyes the freedom to move as they want to, and see what happens. Do your eyes jump large distances and take in quite a few words at a time, making your brain function at a high level of integration, or do your eyes prefer to move with a slower integration of the words?

Furthermore, do you savour the words you are reading, with the enjoyment of the words themselves, or are the words simply inanimate tools which you are using to grasp intellectual significance?

All of this relates directly to your basic perceptual habits, to your ability to enjoy the act of seeing, and your potential for visual growth and expansion. There is certainly nothing wrong with reading at breakneck pace if you are needing to gain a quick overview, or if what you are reading does not deeply concern you.

But now that you are turning to explore your own visual experience, to what extent do your eyes want to slow down and take a deeper look at what is going by?

You will notice that we are talking about your eyes as if they were independent beings, but in reality, we are talking about the entire visual system which makes up your experience of seeing. Seeing is actually an act of the entire mind, body, and soul, when given the chance. When we talk about allowing your eyes to look at what they want to, we are talking about that entire spontaneous being which lives deep within you, which was punished and conditioned and inhibited into retreat long ago, but which is still there, waiting for a friendly nod of recognition and acceptance.

MUSCULAR CO-ORDINATION

So with this understanding of the depths we are talking about, we can now begin to approach the actual ways in which your eyes function. We are going to talk about muscles which surround your eyes, for instance. They are called the extraocular eye muscles, and we might as well call them by their medical name, so you will know what a doctor is talking about if you have extraocular eye troubles in the future, or if your child has such troubles.

But let's consider these muscles first of all without any mention of troubles. Let's see them as great athletes, working constantly, with almost no word of thanks, to point both eyes in the same direction, so that you can see what is in front of you clearly.

This ability to point both eyes at a single point in space, and to move both eyes together to look at the next words or object, is a remarkable physiological/cognitive feat. Six muscles in each eye work together to move the eyes in their sockets, with the brain directing the entire show.

We should move back to the early months of childhood in order to follow the development of this ability.

Very early in your life, while your brain was still in the physical process of developing towards mature functioning, you began

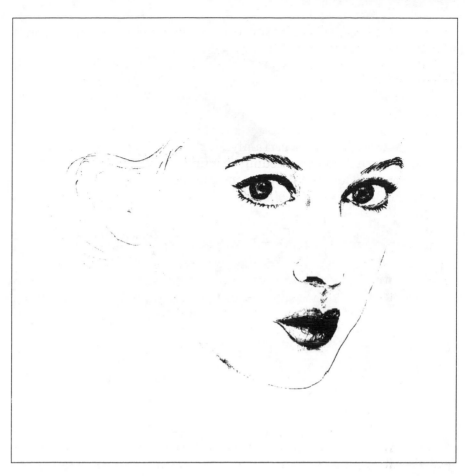

exploring your visual potential. After being born, you stared out at the strange blurry realms which surrounded you, and inherent systems inside you began to take in the visual stimuli and process them.

At first, your eye muscles had almost no co-ordination. You stared randomly at whatever might be in front of you, absorbing passively the world around you.

But quite quickly, your brain's natural curiosity to see the outside world stimulated the learning process which matched muscular performance with the result of co-ordinated looking. You turned your head in the direction of your mother's voice, and found out that you could also just turn your eyes without turning your head, to look in different directions.

Soon you could follow the movement of objects around the room, and your brain continued to process the vast amount of visual information it was receiving moment to moment through each day, until a coherent image of the outside world also existed inside your head.

7

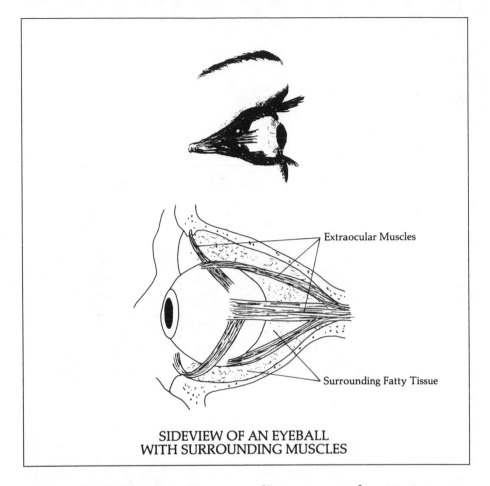

Extraocular Muscles

Surrounding Fatty Tissue

SIDEVIEW OF AN EYEBALL
WITH SURROUNDING MUSCLES

Not only did the muscles surrounding your eyes learn to turn your eyes together to look at different objects. Other muscles, inside the eye itself, learned to tense and relax in order to shift the focus of your inner lens from near to far, and back to near again. This focusing from near to far is called accommodation, and it is the other primary muscular performance which makes clear, efficient, relaxed seeing possible.

The muscles which control your ability to focus from near to far are called the ciliary muscles. The important point to remember is that when they contract and are tense, they alter the shape of the inner lens so that you can see objects up close. When the ciliary muscles relax, the lens flattens so that you can see objects in the distance.

As you are reading this book, your ciliary muscles are in constant contraction, working hard to maintain the up-close focus required for reading. In contrast, pause a moment and look off into the distance beyond the book.

Your brain, naturally, is in control of the tensing and relaxing of the

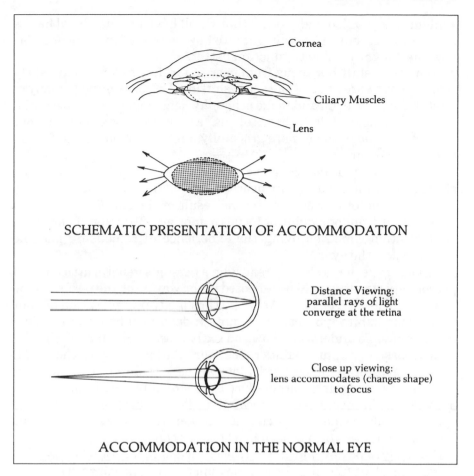

SCHEMATIC PRESENTATION OF ACCOMMODATION

Distance Viewing:
parallel rays of light
converge at the retina

Close up viewing:
lens accommodates (changes shape)
to focus

ACCOMMODATION IN THE NORMAL EYE

ciliary muscles, as well as of the muscles surrounding the eyes (called the extraocular muscles). It is the co-ordination of your inner intentions and wishes, with the performance of your visual muscles, which determines where in space you are going to focus at any given moment. For instance, right now, you are choosing mentally to focus up-close on this page, and your brain is sending constantly-changing orders to the eye muscles to make the act of reading this page possible.

We take all of this for granted, and allow the process to function unconsciously most of the time. But the simple visual act of reading is quite remarkable.

INDIVIDUAL HABITS

If we remember that visual functioning is dependent on muscular performance, we can see how each of us will have a somewhat different way of looking. In the same way that each of us learned to walk in a unique manner, each of us also learned to move the eyes and to focus in a unique manner. To understand that we all have unique visual habits is to gain an essential first insight into how our eyes function, and also how they might be able to function better.

Some of us shift our focus from near to far, for instance, extremely rapidly, not aware at all of the act of shifting. In the same way, many of us stand up, sit down, and make other physical movements with rapid, jerky motions, while others of us are more conscious of our movements, make them more gracefully, and in fact enjoy the feeling of the movement.

What about you and your eye movements? Are you aware of the shifting of your focus from near to far, or do you block out this movement and only focus on the end result of the shift? Are you in a hurry to get from one point of focus to another, or do you make these shifts 'within time', enjoying the experience of refocusing and the movement of the eyes?

As you are perhaps already realizing, a person's general attitude and personality structure will be reflected in the way he or she performs the visual shifting movements. As we go through this exploration of your own seeing habits, you can gain quite a deep insight into your own inner nature. To understand how you see is to see yourself more clearly.

Obviously, our visual habits reflect our relationship with the world. Some people, for instance, hardly look at the outside world at all. They have habits of staring, rather than habits of constantly moving the eyes to take in more visual information. The natural tendency of the eyes is to shift the point of focus regularly, so that every second a new bit of the outside world is seen by the inner consciousness.

But many of us developed habits early in childhood, or when we first began school, of freezing the eye movements so that very little visual information was received by the brain. In fact, this is one of the most common habits we have in our culture these days which reduces our interaction with the outside world and thus reduces our ability to live in it successfully.

Why would such a habit develop?

As I mentioned in the introduction, we cannot separate the physiological from the psychological aspects of seeing. The way our muscular system functions is so intimately related to the way our emotions function, that they must be taken as an organic whole, indivisible in everyday life. If you have the visual habit of staring, of not regularly shifting your focus to give your brain more information about the outside worked, then something must have happened to you in your childhood to make you avoid behaviour which brought you more intimately into contact with your environment.

If you have a habit of not taking in much visual information, you must have, at some point, not wanted to see what was around you.

Conversely, if you have healthy habits of enjoying the visual environment you are in, your early years must have been blessed with the harmony and security which encourages such an openness to the outside world.

Consider an infant who is just learning how to see. Imagine that the emotional atmosphere in the home is full of anger, arguments, grief. The parents are fighting, perhaps they are in the process of separating, and the baby is caught in the middle of an anxious, angry battle of the sexes.

The baby will respond to this turmoil with fright, naturally. Its own security is threatened by the instability of the parents, and so a general state of fear will pervade the baby's body. This is an extreme situation, offered so that we can clearly see how the emotional environment affects the visual habits.

The baby will be frightened of the outside world if it is loud, violent, anxious, unloving. Instead of the early experience of seeing being enjoyable exploration, secure and inviting, the outside world will appear threatening, dangerous, something to be avoided.

So as the brain learns to direct the eye muscles to look, the emotional atmosphere will affect this learning with an avoidance pattern. Simple shifting of focus from near to far will be influenced by what the baby sees when it looks in the distance. If such looking becomes associated with experiences of fear and tension, then distance focusing will be impaired.

Another fascinating aspect of seeing has to do with the actual experience of shifting from looking at one object, to another object. If we feel comfortable in our environment, if we have not developed a fear of what we might encounter in the outside world, then the act of looking in a new direction, to see what new visual experience we might encounter, is a pleasurable, even exciting activity. The world is always interesting and stimulating, as we regularly shift our focus to see what changes might be occurring around us.

But for many of us, change is associated with an uncertain, insecure, even negative expectation. Especially in early childhood, if we had many experiences of shifting our focus and encountering something which frightened us, we came to associate such visual movements with apprehension, not with anticipation. And therefore, we tended to inhibit eye movement. As an avoidance of negative experience, we habitually reduced our intake of new visual scenes.

Growing up is a mixed blessing for everyone. There is always a certain amount of trauma, apprehension, and anxiety in childhood. Each of us reacted to our own traumas with our own contractions and avoidance patterns. One question of this book is focused on how such experiences might have negatively altered your visual functioning, and more importantly how you can now begin to move beyond those old visual habits, so that your overall experience of seeing is more enjoyable and efficient.

Let's begin with a simple yet revealing exercise. Below is a large circle. As you approach this circle visually, remain aware of how in fact you look at it. Take a relaxed breath and spend the next six breaths, or about half a minute, looking at the circle, noticing what your eyes naturally tend to do when looking at such a visual stimulus. Be open to whatever discoveries you might make regarding your habits of seeing.

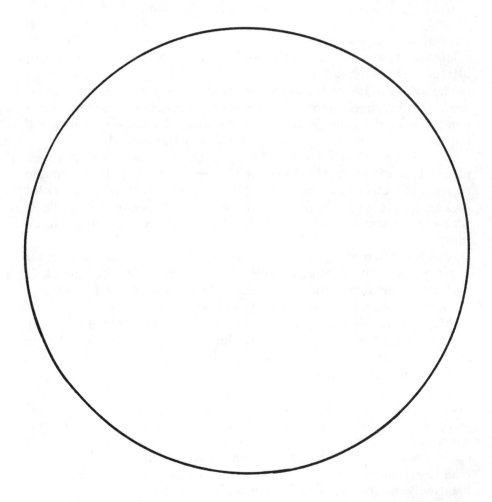

Some people prefer to stare at the centre of the circle, allowing their peripheral vision to take in the whole circle at once. Some people tend to look all round the circle, with quick eye movements which cover the entire distance of the curved line so that the eyes move around and make their own circular movement.

Did you notice how your breathing was affected by the task (or pleasure) of looking at the circle? Another primary factor in seeing is the way we breath when performing different visual functions. Our breathing is a direct barometer of our inner feelings. If we are relaxed and enjoying the experience of looking at something, our breathing is smooth, full, and rhythmic. Our visual habits tend to match our breathing habits, and so we can use conscious awareness and alterations in our breathing habits to improve our visual habits as well. They go together.

If looking at the circle generated an old inhibition in your breathing, because you felt you had somehow to perform as you were forced to do at school, then your visual habits were also certainly affected. At the same time that you turned your attention to the circle, part of you also wanted to avoid the experience altogether. So as you looked at the circle, you might have felt a conflict.

This conflict is crucial to vision impairment. If you force your eyes to perform a visual task, but at the same time would prefer to avoid the task, the resultant conflict causes tension throughout the visual system.

Let's return to the circle, and explore your own unconscious visual habits in more depth. This time, the circle is divided into four quadrants (see page 14). Notice as you slowly move your eyes around each quadrant, which one is easiest to follow, and which one is most difficult. Watch your breathing throughout!

Was your breathing smooth as you followed the outer perimeter of the circle, of did it tend to freeze at times, to become irregular and tense in the chest?

Did you notice if there was a relationship between your eye movements and your breathing?

Almost all of us have particular regions of a circle where we enjoy movement and 'feel' of our eyes, and certain regions of the circle where our breathing becomes tense and we experience poorly co-ordinated visual movement.

The emotional, psychoanalytical reasons for such reactions to a simple circle are fascinating but complex. For our purposes in this book, it is enough to realize consciously what habits we have in the act of seeing. Then we can begin to alter the habits. Through exploring the physical habit, we often resolve old fears and conditioned expectations as well.

At this point in the book, it is time to bring attention to bear on a basic visual habit which you might want to change. You have been reading this book, focusing up close, for quite some time now. Your ciliary muscles have been under constant tension, in order to focus your lenses up-close for reading. This tension should be relieved periodically, or chronic tension can be developed in the ciliary muscles, inhibiting your ability to shift your focus into the distance.

So a good habit is as follows. Every twenty pages of reading should be followed by a six-breath break, where you look off into the distance (even five feet is good) and relax the eye muscles for just half a minute. Try this now!

ACCOMMODATION AND TRACKING

We have now taken a first look at the two main muscular activities of the eyes, the act of shifting focus from near to far (accommodation) and the act of moving the eyes to follow a moving object or to shift to another object (tracking).

Your ability to perform these two actions is a variable which can be improved. Simple but powerful exercises can be performed regularly if you want to enhance your visual performance.

For instance, with accommodation, you can actually improve your focal shifting every time you consciously notice that you are making this shift throughout every day. The act of being aware of how you perform focal shifting, brings the conscious brain into play in evaluating your habitual functioning, and making corrections where needed.

Conscious awareness is in fact one of the primary tools for visual improvement. First you must be aware of your old habits. Then you must allow alterations in those habits. By bringing the attention of the brain to focus on your vision habits, the brain naturally goes to work to maximize performance. Our basic problem is that we remain unconscious of our habits, and thus function only according to previous programming.

So new learning can take place every time you are aware of shifting from near to far, and back to near again. You can see how smooth and relaxed the shifting is, and encourage improvement.

However, a word of caution. When you begin watching yourself and observing your vision habits, be sure not to instantly judge your habits as 'bad' or 'wrong'. As soon as you reject your present functioning, you lose touch with the natural process which will improve that functioning. The process of visual recovery, on all levels, requires an attitude of acceptance and self-love, not of rejection and separation.

This is not a philosophical aspect of visual recovery. We are talking about your attitude towards your eyes. If you accept them as they are, your brain can then make the first small step in growth, allowing your habits to shift slightly in healthy directions.

But if you reject your habit, a serious psychological separation takes place. You have nothing to build upon but your existing habits and performance. If you reject that habit, no growth can take place.

At the heart of this growth is the fact that your brain knows how healthy vision functions. You were born with a natural ability to see clearly. The distortions of your seeing, unless caused by strong genetic misfortune, came about through emotional and environmental stress which caused a variation away from clear efficient seeing. You now want to activate the natural functioning. And to do this, you must begin with where you are, and step by step evolve towards more spontaneous, natural seeing. The key word is evolve. Evolution only takes place through acceptance of the present condition.

So regardless of your present habits or visual dysfunction, you can improve this basic functioning of the eyes called accommodation. If you have clear physical eyesight, or if you are near or far-sighted, the exercise is equally important, and provides a building block for future exercises.

1. Hold one finger up fairly close to your eyes, perhaps six inches from your nose as shown in the illustration.
2. Hold the finger of the other hand up in the distance, so that you can shift your focus from one to the other.
3. Choose a third point of focus further in the distance, which you can shift to beyond the second finger.
4. With every inhalation and exhalation, shift your focus from one point to the next. Match smooth breathing with smooth focal shifting.

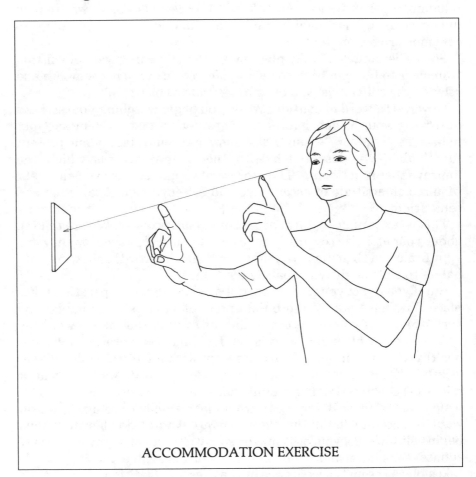

ACCOMMODATION EXERCISE

Do this for perhaps ten full cycles. Notice that awareness of your breathing is the active ingredient which makes this exercise potent. Through being aware of both your breathing and your eyes at the same time, you integrate your emotions, your physical functioning, and your visual functioning. So in all vision exercises, remember to be aware of your breathing!

You will find that when you shift your focus from one point to the other as fast as possible, you tend to freeze your breathing. Speed is not the goal in this exercise. Conscious awareness of the muscles making the shift is the goal. Once this conscious awareness is gained, your brain is in a position to improve its normally unconscious activities.

Habits are curious things. Their purpose is to help us function in an existing environment, and the form they take depends on our conditioning at the time. At first they are conscious, but gradually they become unconscious, not directly influenced by changing environments.

This means that old habits can get in our way if we find ourselves in new situations which are better suited to different behaviour. To change old habits to more appropriate ones, we need first to regain our awareness of their patterns, and then to learn new variations on them.

The faster we perform a movement, the harder it is to be conscious of it. Sudden movements cannot be followed by our consciousness. Only when we slow down the movement, can we be aware of it 'in time'. With accommodation, the slower you shift from one point to the other, the more clearly you can feel the muscular shifting inside the eyes – and the more quickly your brain can begin to direct that muscular habit towards smoother, more relaxed functioning. Especially with myopia and presbyopia (near-sightedness and far-sightedness) this awareness is critical.

BLINKING

Another factor which we should begin to be aware of is blinking. The eyes naturally blink, in order to maintain proper lubrication of the surface of the eyes (conjunctiva) and also in order to give the retina a moment's rest, to temporarily stop the flow of information to the brain, much as a comma or a full-stop temporarily stops the flow of words and ideas on a page.

Blinking can also be affected by emotions. People who are frightened of letting go, of leaving the known and venturing into the unknown, tend to blink less often than people who welcome an end of one period and a beginning of another.

What about you? As you are reading this line of words, are you aware of your blinking? Do you punctuate every few lines with a blink, or do you tend to stare without blinking for longer periods of time?

Some people blink very rapidly, as if frightened of losing contact with the outside world. Other people blink very slowly, as if savouring their inner worlds and providing a balance between inner and outer awareness. What do you do, right now?

When you talk to people, notice how they blink. It is fascinating to see how you are affected when someone blinks slowly while talking to you, as opposed to staring constantly at you with no blinking and no relief from contact. To become aware of these habits is to open up a new realm. Normal blinking occurs every five to ten seconds. But we should not establish rigid rules. What do you prefer?

PERFORMANCE EXERCISES

Our ability to shift our eyes from one object to another, or from one point of a picture to another, can be enhanced quickly and dramatically. There is no reason for us to hang on to old habits which keep us sluggish, inhibited, slow learners and unresponsive participants in life.

As with your physical body in general, increased muscle tone, strength, and co-ordination come about through conscious exercise, deeper awareness of movement, and the integration of mental and physiological functioning. The eyes, like any other part of the body, will respond to increased attention.

Whether we are driving a car and looking for red lights while also watching out for the cyclist in our rear-view mirror, or doing anything else which requires the regular observation of more than one point in space, we are performing an athletic feat. Our breathing is the first factor to consider. If we are tense or anxious, our breathing will be shallow and irregular, interfering with oxygen intake and mental concentration, as well as visual performance.

Once the awareness of breathing is achieved, the next step is to integrate this breath awareness with visual awareness. If you are conscious of the shifts your eyes are making, this shifting can be done with less tension, which means more smoothly, and with more co-ordination.

Look at the circle opposite. Shift from one section of the circle to the next with matching breathing, allowing your eyes to move along the curved line between the markers. Notice the feeling in your eyes as you do this seemingly simple visual exercise.

A few years ago, while developing a similar vision programme for the America Airline Pilots' Association, I was struck by the improvement which was possible, over a short period of time, in visual performance. Even pilots who had been flying commercial jets for twenty years could enhance their visual potential through becoming conscious of old habits which got in the way of smooth movements.

For instance, one pilot had flown jets in Vietnam as his first professional experience. Naturally, the emotional tensions, however well hidden at the time, generated tensions in the visual apparatus as well. If you expect to be blown out of the air at any moment by an

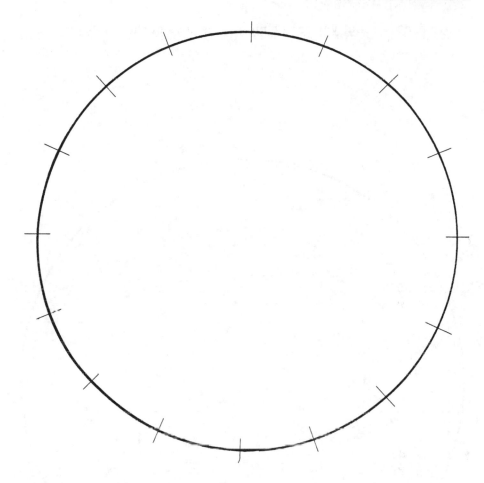

enemy aircraft, your breathing and visual performance are going to be more tense than if you are flying quietly over the Grand Canyon.

Only when the old habits of tension are experienced consciously can they begin to be reversed. So notice your breathing as you do this next exercise, for which you will need to look at the circle on page 20. Simply start counting from one to twenty or fifty, and with each number you say to yourself, shift your eyes to a new target, randomly. With every five counts, shift your breathing from inhale to exhale and back. You will be taking a picture once a second with this exercise, which is a good rate for the brain to process visual information. Just see how you enjoy functioning at this optimum level of visual performance. Try it now.

For a more specific 'tracking' exercise, look from one point to the next, counting to six points in the inhale, then six points on the following exhale, through six breath cycles. Allow your eyes to move randomly to different dots as they prefer. See if you can be aware of the visual experience of jumping from one dot to another – slow down the

19

movements so that you can be more conscious of the whole process.

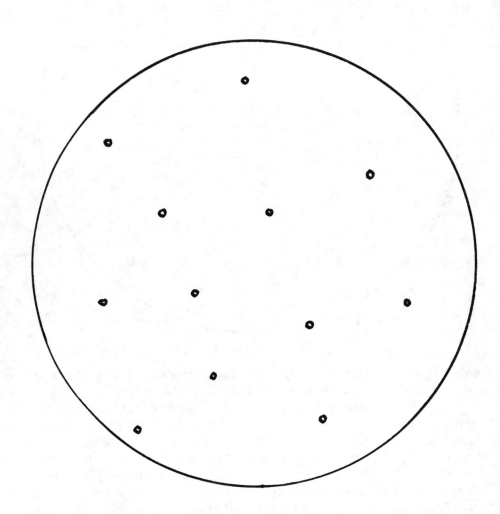

For a variation of this 'tracking' exercise, you might enjoy the following movements of the eyes as you let your visual attention move along the lines. Inhaling for three lines, and then exhaling for three lines, might be your preferred breathing/seeing rhythm, but feel free to explore different breathing rates.

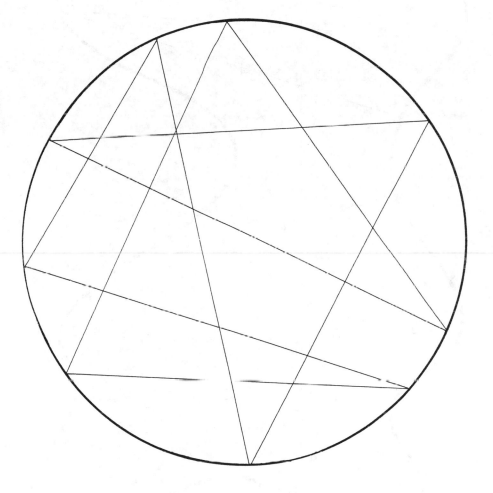

Follow the curved outer line as if you were driving around a race track. Then feel the mental shift as you change to the straight lines inside, breathing smoothly through the choices of direction.

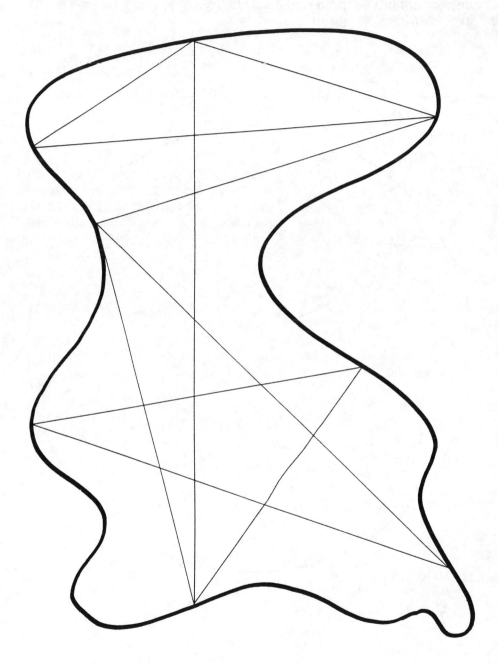

PALMING

To finish this chapter, we should introduce the basic eye relaxation exercise. After doing such exercises as the last one, you should give your eyes a total break from the 'work' of looking. The best way to do this is as follows:

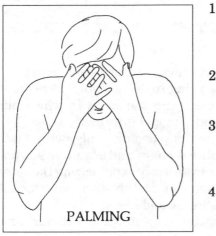

PALMING

1. Stand or sit quietly as shown in the illustration, and cover one eye with one hand, the other eye with the other hand.
2. Cup your palm slightly so that it is right over the closed eye, but not touching it.
3. Your fingers should overlap on your forehead with your thumbs on your temples and your little fingers on either side of the nose.
4. Relax your neck and lower your head, so that your arms are relaxed down to your sides as shown in the illustration.
5. Concentrate on your breathing, and then expand your awareness to include your eyes themselves.
6. You might want to repeat the word 'relax' each time you inhale and exhale, to further generate total relaxation, both in the eyes, the breathing, and the mind itself.

You will find that this posture almost instantly brings relief from visual tension, and also encourages general relaxation and peace. Do it often!

2 · EXPANDING OUR PERCEPTION

We have thus far focused our discussion on the actual muscular performance of the eyes. We are now going to delve a step deeper into our visual functioning, through considering the ways in which our brains use the eyes to collect meaningful visual information.

When we 'conceive' something, we are dealing only with inner conceptual levels of our minds, with pure thought and cognitive images. But when we 'perceive' something, we are directly experiencing the outer world. Our perceptual habits are as unique as our speaking voice or our thumbprints, although not as easy to locate and identify.

Also, our perceptual habits are subject to emotional distortions, confusion, laziness, and inflexibility. Our overall experience and success throughout our lives is strongly determined and limited by our perceptual habits. In fact, much of the visual distortion associated with myopia is generated not by incorrect focusing, but by other perceptual habits. And even people with perfectly clear physical vision often demonstrate great weaknesses in perceptual habits.

To understand clearly the basic ingredients of perception, we need to begin with an exploration of the connection between the eyes and the brain.

THE EYE-BRAIN CONNECTION

We tend to think of the eyes as isolated organs, quite separate from the brain itself. But in reality the eyes are a direct outgrowth of the brain, with millions of brain cells existing in the retina of each eye. These cells are specialized brain tissue which are photosensitive, or sensitive to light. Their job is to receive the incoming light, to codify it into simple meaningful units, and then to send this information to the brain.

Recent research has shown that babies are born with only partially developed retinas. In the same way that the brain itself continues to develop after birth, the retinal cells establish a complex computer network amongst themselves, in response to the visual inputs of early childhood.

Thus, a child with a visually stimulating environment will develop

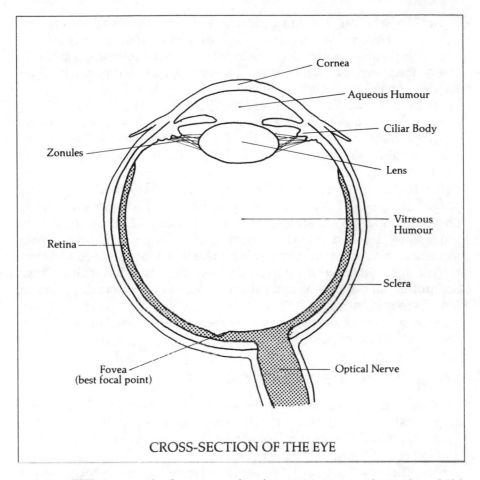

Cornea

Aqueous Humour

Ciliar Body

Zonules

Lens

Vitreous
Humour

Retina

Sclera

Fovea
(best focal point)

Optical Nerve

CROSS-SECTION OF THE EYE

quite a different retinal communications system to that of a child locked away in a blank room, with very little human interaction or visual contact with movement and form.

At one time it was thought that the retinas in the back of the eyes simply received visual information like camera film, and then sent that information off to the brain for analysis. But in fact, the retina itself makes the first steps in the interpretation of the visual inputs, and then sends its interpretation off to the brain for further analysis, labelling, association with past inputs, and image formation.

Whether you like the idea or are bothered by the limitations implied, your early childhood visual experiences did at least partly determine your present perception ability.

When visual information comes flooding into the eyes, and lands (hopefully in focus) on the surface of the retina, the millions of photosensitive cells give basically very simple yes–no responses. Primarily, the retina works to detect differences in intensities of light.

It notices whether a shadow exists, where brightness changes into darkness. This creates the basic black and white image of vision.

One step more advanced, the cells in the eyes detect variations in the colour frequencies of light, so that we can tell the difference between shades of red, blue, yellow, and so on.

With this simple computer analysis of the incoming light, assumptions are then made about what is being seen. Groups of cells join together to make generalizations about where shadow begins, and where brightness begins. This is the beginning of a meaningful image, which we call form.

The brain is not passive in the seeing process. It is actively seeking particular types of information, depending on the emotional mood, physical imperatives, and mental expectancies. Depending on the immediate interest of the person, the mind processes visual information in different ways, taking the basic images received from the retinas, and integrating this immediate information with the vast computer-bank of past visual information, in order to make meaning out of the perception.

What we actually experience as seeing is the end result of a highly complex process of perception.

FOUR TYPES OF PERCEPTION

In order to expand our perceptual habits, we need first to see consciously how the brain naturally goes about gathering information. There are four different types of perception, and we can separate them and experience each of them – right now.

First there is the natural tendency to perceive movement. This is a powerful instinctual factor in human survival, a genetic endowment derived from many millions of years of primitive life on planet Earth. We seek and detect movement, especially when we feel endangered, or are in a 'hunting' state of mind.

Right now, look up from the book if you want, and experience this tendency for yourself. Just look around you, with the sole purpose of detecting movement. Stay aware of your breathing as you do this, and observe how natural it is to focus at this level of perception.

You can feel how this perceptual focus on movement illicits a general feeling in the body, one related to physical readiness.

The second basic element of perception has to do with the inherent tendency of the brain to seek out form in the visual inputs it receives. Whenever we look at something, we naturally try to find a form in the immediate perception which reminds us of previous similar forms. In this way, we find meaning in what we see, based on past experience.

The perception of form is an active movement of the eyes, following lines, curves, shadows, and angles, and sending this information to the brain for analysis. Notice that the word 'in-form-ation' itself conveys this basic nature of form in human understanding.

Pause and experience this distinct functioning of your perceptual system. Look around you, but this time simply look to see form. Run your eyes along lines and curves, take in the perimeter of objects, the shape and structure.

The natural tendency of the brain to seek out form is accompanied by its own emotional and mental state, which you can feel for yourself through such focusing and eye movement. Notice if your breathing tends to freeze, or to remain even, as you explore the dimensions of your environment.

After movement and form, we find a third natural dimension of perception. This is the realm of colour perception. The eyes have two different types of retinal cells – the cones which detect colour, and the rods, which only detect black and white. During the daytime when lighting is sufficient, the cones are stimulated for very detailed perception. At night, when there isn't enough light to detect colour, the rods come into action, giving us at least limited vision.

So we have two separate visual experiences, one in the daytime (colour perception) and quite a different one at night (black and white perception). Right at dusk, when we are shifting from cones to rods, we often feel visually confused and uncertain, as you perhaps have noticed. The shift from colour to black and white changes our whole 'feel' for the world outside.

Colour is an inherent aspect of life on planet Earth. It is an expression of the basic vibratory nature of the universe. And as we take in different colours from our environment, we are sending to the brain an infinite variety of vibrational stimulation. Researchers studying the effects of colour on the brain are still only beginning to explore the subject, but it is obvious that different colours do have different impacts on our consciousness and general functioning.

Look around you for six breaths or more right now, and just look to see colour, nothing else. Absorb all the colours you encounter, and see what you 'feel' from each colour.

We now come to a final aspect of perception, one which is often overlooked. Along with movement, form, and colour, we also look in order to perceive space. This is quite a different mode of looking, because we are not looking 'at' anything at all; instead, we are looking to experience the actual volume of our surroundings, the air itself.

This perception is intimately related both to superior physical performance, as with great athletes, and also to expanded states of spiritual perception, as described by the great mystics throughout the ages. Unfortunately, the loss of the perception of space is associated with mental illness, anxiety, stress, and any condition of fear.

Look around you one more time, and this time, look at nothing in particular. Stare into space, and hold your focus on your breathing at the same time, to enhance this perception. Feel the volume of the surroundings, and notice how you feel while your perception is thus focused. Try this exercise now.

The illustration opposite gives a direct guide for the perception of space, or volume. This type of perception is often in need of considerable help in order for its natural potential to be encouraged.

Simply stare at the centre of this circle, while expanding your awareness to include the outer perimeter of the circle as well, so that you see the entire area inside the circle 'at once'.

You perhaps noticed that this 'space perception' encourages quite a different state of consciousness to that generated by the other three modes of seeing. With movement and form, the eyes are very busy focusing on particular points in space, and looking from one point in space to another. This active way of looking involves precision functioning, and also tends to exclude from consciousness everything in the visual field except the point of attention at the moment.

Quite conversely, when we look just to experience colour, we expand our perceptual field of attention to include the general area which is a particular colour. Thus, colour perception is a less precise visual function than form and movement perception. As would be expected, research has found different regions in the brain associated with these different visual functions. To perceive colour is to be in a different mental state to that in which we perceive movement, or form.

When we advance to the perception of volume, of space, we encounter the opposite extreme to movement perception. We find the eyes not moving at all, the focal point expanded to include the entire visual field, and the state of mind alert but not active with analysis of specific visual data.

In fact, with the perception of space, we find a state of mind conducive to meditation, intuitive reflection, and a focusing of the mind's attention on the integration of the outside world with the inside world, without differentiation. The breathing relaxes , the eye muscles also relax, and heart rate slows down.

The principal concern at this point has to do with your habitual visual patterns. Some of us have a tendency to be lost much of the time in the meditative, unfocused perception of space. Conversely, some of us are so concerned with our survival, with anxieties and anticipations of danger, that we are overly focused on the perception of movement, looking all the time for a visual input which we should react to.

There are those of us who are chronically focused on form, looking to make meaning of everything around us, wanting to form concrete mental images of our environment so that we have it somehow 'under our control'. And finally there are those of us who love colour, who enjoy spending considerable time each day just absorbing beautiful scenes, watching the leaves on a tree, or gazing into a sunset.

What about you?

Begin to notice, moment to moment, how you are spending your visual days.

There is no 'right' or 'wrong' way to perceive the world around you. But there are appropriate times for being alert for movement, and other times when aesthetic appreciation is called for.

A healthy balance of all four modes of perception should be the goal. This means that you should consciously spend more time exploring whichever mode of perception you tend to avoid. Give yourself one-minute exercises once an hour, focusing for just six breaths on the two modes you tend to avoid. This conscious action is your tool to expanded perception.

You might find that your habits of perception are very deeply ingrained in your personality. People with difficulties in perceiving volume, for instance, are usually so caught up in the game of survival that they never take the time to relax and simply enjoy their environment. They keep themselves so busy in their heads, with plans for the future and concepts about their present situation, that their consciousness is collapsed to the centre of their cognitive mind, rather than expanded to include their surroundings. In extreme cases of this fixation on form and movement, chronic anxiety states and stress patterns erode both physical and mental health.

For these people, simple perceptual expansion exercises are often extremely helpful. By learning to shift the visual focus to include the immediate surroundings, the colours and volume of the room, a positive shift in emotional and mental states is induced. The expansion of consciousness is generated through expansion of perception. This is an old spiritual trick of yogis and primitive societies as well, and you can use it to your advantage if you feel the need.

Conversely, for those of us who are overly fixated on expansive, unfocused states, simple exercising of the form and movement perception abilities of the mind will help to shift habits in more functional, active directions. Increasing eye movement, co-ordinated with breath awareness, can evoke powerful changes in our behaviour and personality profiles. The choice, of course, is always yours.˙

The goal of such perception exercises should be a functional integration of the four modes of seeing, so that you are looking to see all four dimensions together. This is a habit you can develop. All it requires is conscious exercising of the four modes, one after the other, with each visual focus you encounter.

For instance, as you look at this page, you can first notice that there is no movement (detecting no movement is the same process as detecting movement, by the way). Then you can instantly shift from movement to form, and scan the page to see what general lines and structures you detect, what groupings of words, what blank spaces, and so forth. Then you can look to detect colour, and determine that there is only black and white. And finally, you can be aware of the space between your eyes and the page, and the space which surrounds the book.

Thus, in a very brief time, you have covered all four parameters of perception, and know that you have a complete visual experience.

It is helpful to pair the words with the visual focus. Memorize 'movement', 'form', 'colour', and 'volume'. Then you can think each word in turn, and your mind will quickly learn to match the word with the perceptual mode.

I find it most helpful to match each word with a breath, so that your awareness of your whole being is enhanced as you go through the four modes of seeing.

With the first word, 'movement', your eyes will instantly start scanning your environment, detecting movement or the lack of it. Then this aspect can rest, as you go on to 'form', which is also active eye movement, returning to the same visual field that you scanned for movement, but looking instead for meaningful patterns and structures.

You can see that, survival-wise, there is a natural order to these four perceptual modes. First, it might be essential to detect anything moving – this instinct is so deep that it is vital to include it in any vision-improvement work. Then a more thorough viewing of the scene is called for, to determine what is actually being looked at, based on past experience.

And then, the experience is not complete without taking in colour, enjoying the sensation of the different qualities of light vibrations as they enter your being through your eyes. As you say 'colour', hold this general word in your mind, so that you don't become busy labelling each colour by its name. This returns you to the 'form' mode of analysis, rather than direct experiencing of colour.

Finally, as you hold the word 'volume' or 'space' in your mind, you allow a further expansion to occur, as you take in 'everything at once' and gain an intuitive contact with the relationship between your presence and the surroundings. With this final step, you contain the full experience of your surroundings, a total perception.

Perceptual Integration

- One breath for 'movement'.
- One breath for 'form'.
- One breath for 'colour'.
- One breath for 'volume'.

Apply this formula of perception to any object. Fully focus on the particular mode of perception you are saying to yourself for one breath. Then let go of this focus completely, and turn to the next mode.

When you have taken in each of the four modes, continue to look at the object as you breath for two final breaths, experiencing the integration of the four modes of perception.

If you do this exercise ten times a day (which is only five minutes total time) you will powerfully enhance your perceptual habits.

3 · VISUALIZATION: THE EYES AND THE MIND

Once we have received the visual inputs which give us the experience of 'seeing' something, further perception habits determine how well we hold that image in our mind, and to what extent we really saw the image in various parts of our minds.

Some of us are naturally good at visualizing what we have seen in the past, whether it be a moment ago or a decade ago. Others of us have serious difficulties even in looking at a face or object and then closing our eyes and visualizing what we just saw.

To a certain extent this ability seems related to our different genetic endowments of mental functioning. But emotional trauma is also a primary factor in the inability to visualize. We have remarkable powers to block from consciousness things which we do not want to remember. Unfortunately, when we block one memory, we tend to block a complete assortment of related memories as well.

Thus, if you were 4 years old and were confronted with the threatening face of someone who scared you deeply, you might try to blot the memory of this face from your mind. In so doing, you might develop a block against remembering any face at all. This is a very common psychological phenomenon.

Regardless of psychoanalytical explanations, we can progress with exploring your current habits of visualization, and offer guidelines for consciously beginning to improve these habits. Regardless of your visual condition, this level of vision improvement is valuable.

VISUALIZATION OF FORM

First of all, take a quick look at the picture opposite, for just one breath, and then close your eyes and see how well the picture remains in your inner mind's eye.

For some of you, that was easy; you could close your eyes and see all the lines at once, as a complete visual image. For others of you, it was difficult or seemingly impossible. So now you know where you stand, with regards to simple non-emotive visualization. Regardless of your current ability, I assure you that you can increase this ability considerably, and encourage this development.

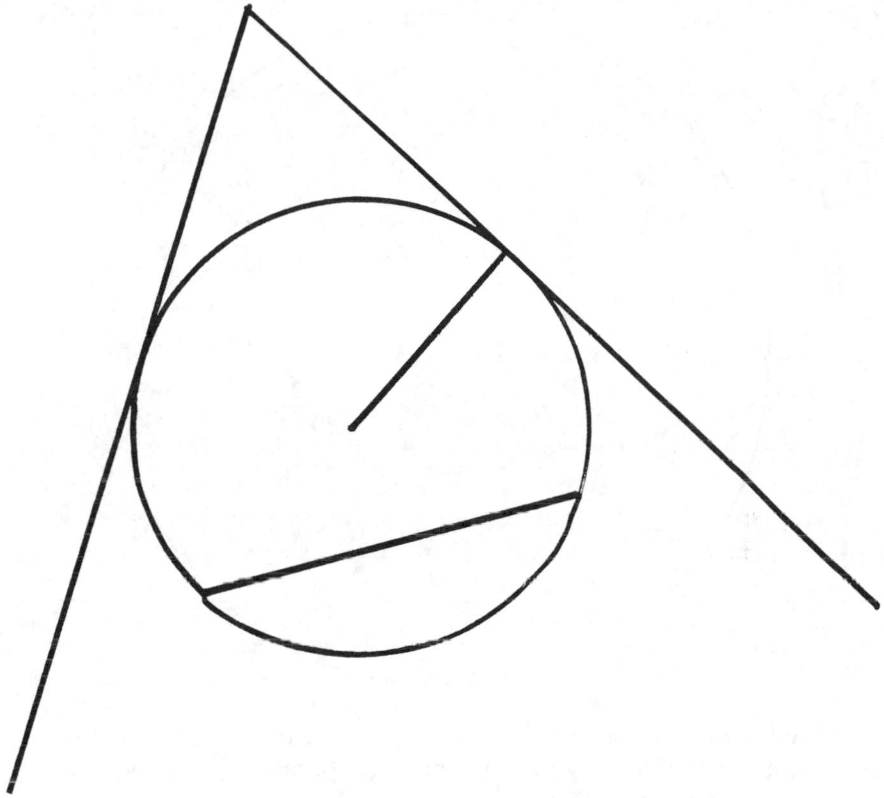

To see your basic patterns for visualization, let's return to a more simple image. Look at the circle on the next page, and then close your eyes and see what remains in your mind's eye:

Try this again: look for one breath, without 'trying' to remember the circle at all. Just look as you breathe. Then close your eyes, breathe another breath, and effortlessly look to see what remains in your inner mind's eye.

You will find that conscious awareness of your breathing tends to enhance visualization. This is because your breath is linked to emotional conditioning, and by consciously recognizing this dimension, you do not fall victim to unconscious anxieties related to visualization.

Almost all of us associate visualizing with fear. This is because we had to memorize images in school, and were under pressure of punishment or ridicule if we couldn't recall the image successfully.

Unfortunately, fear is the great destroyer of such abilities as visualization. If you are frightened that you might not succeed in remembering a visual image, you reduce your ability to remember.

So an elementary trick with visualization improvement is to put

33

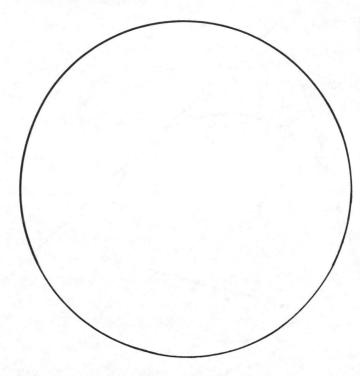

your focus first on your breathing, to allow it to become relaxed and smooth, and then while you maintain this breath awareness, look at what you want to visualize.

Try this again – each time you turn your focus to consciously exploring this visualization process, you are improving that ability. Take a deep breath, exhale completely, and then as you inhale air, inhale the circle also:

Now close your eyes and visualize each of the two pictures you have looked at in this chapter.

VISUALIZATION OF MOVEMENT

Now let's see how you do with the visualization of movement. In a moment, I want you to close your eyes, and imagine that you are watching a bird flying high overhead in a clear sky, soaring with outspread wings in an afternoon breeze. You can tilt your head upwards as if actually watching the great bird, and be sure to remain aware of your breathing as you imagine the powerful, graceful, but unpredictable movement of the bird:

Six breaths of bird-watching exercise

Was that easy, or difficult?

VISUALIZATION OF COLOUR

Next, we are going to explore your ability to imagine colours. Take the colour blue, as the sky was blue when you watched the bird soaring. Just close your eyes and imagine that you are looking at a beautiful, soft, gentle blue sky. Breathe consciously, and take in this colour:

Visualization of the colour blue

VISUALIZATION OF SPACE

Finally, we are going to explore how you relate to the visualization of space. The surroundings you are in right now will serve perfectly. After reading this paragraph, look around you at the volume of the surroundings, as you learned to do in the last chapter. For two breaths, take in the general feeling of space. Then close your eyes, and see how well you can visualize what you just saw, as you continue with your breathing and make no effort:

Visualization of surrounding volume

So now you are beginning to have an idea of your abilities and habits with visualization. The next important step is for you to spend time doing the visualizations which were hard for you. If you want to improve this inner remembrance of what you see, conscious exercising is the path to progress. Notice that you can enjoy this visualization exercising; you can choose to visualize whatever you want, and appreciate the inner images which begin to grow into greater clarity inside you!

There are three final visualizations which we should include in this exploration. First of all, close your eyes for six breaths, and see what visual images come to mind when you focus on how your childhood home looked to you as a boy or girl. Breathe consciously, and be open to whatever visual memories might come to you now:

Visualization of childhood home

Did you notice the relationship between your breathing and the visual memories? To see how breathing and seeing are intimately linked is a major step in perceptual enhancement. If you are locked into unconscious breathing reactions each time you try to visualize something, you will be the prisoner of those habits, and progress will be difficult. But if you begin to observe how your breathing and emotional reactions accompany certain perception tasks, you can consciously grow beyond the old habits.

Now close your eyes and visualize either your father or your mother when you were a child – preferably a real-life visual memory, not a photograph. See how well you can bring such a visual memory into present consciousness. And breathe into whatever emotions might come along with the visualization:

Visualization of parent's face

The final visualization is that of your own face, as you see yourself in the mirror. Close your eyes and simply let your mind's eye remember how you look in the mirror. See how clearly you do look at yourself in the mirror, and if you colour your visualization with emotions, judgements, or distortions. The way you visualize yourself will tell you a great deal about your visualization habits in general. So be honest, be patient, breathe into whatever images come, and allow insights about your visual habits to rise to the surface:

Visualization of your own face

To end this chapter, play with visualizing the following drawing. Allow your eyes to move along all the lines in the drawing, taking in the form. And then stare at the whole picture at once, experiencing the space between you and the picture as well as the image itself. Then close your eyes, see what image remains. Do this several times, and watch the image grow in your mind's eye!

Be sure to include an awareness of your breathing as you do this final exercise. Notice if you give yourself permission to enjoy this exercise, or if you insist on approaching it as 'work'. Visualization is, essentially, a playful sport.

Move your eyes along this racetrack image, enjoying the quick turns and the long stretches of the race. Then just relax and see the whole image at once. Finally, close your eyes and see what image remains in your inner eye. Breathe smoothly!

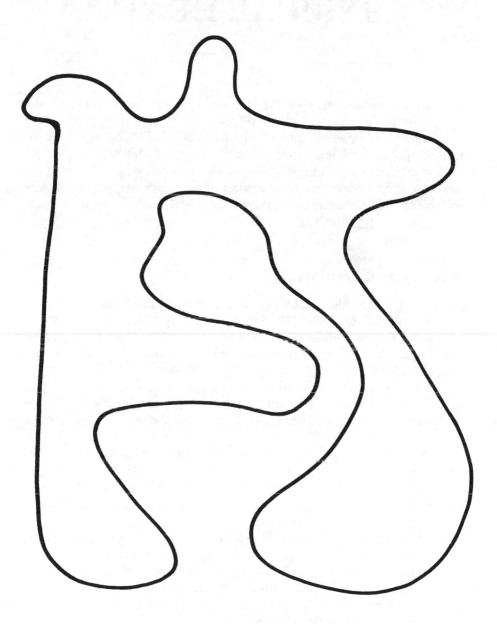

4 · VISUAL HEALTH AND PHYSICAL HEALTH

As long as we see the eyes as isolated sense organs, visual health appears only distantly related to physical health. But the great bulk of medical and psycho-physiological research of the last half-century indicates that our bodies function as an integral whole.

If we look at the health of the eyes in the same way we look at the health of the whole body, we immediately see ways to maximize visual well-being. This chapter will give you general guidelines and specific exercises which optimize physical health as it directly relates to visual functioning.

NOURISHING THE EYES

First of all, we should consider the actual physical make-up of the eyes. Like the rest of the body, the eyes are made up of living tissue which requires regular nutrients to maintain healthy functioning. This means that the food you eat is a factor in your visual health, as it is in overall health.

The cells which make up the eyes are totally dependent on your blood circulation for their very survival. If you exercise regularly and maintain vitality in your body, your eyes will remain dynamic also, well into old age. But if you have poor circulation, eat unbalanced meals, and exercise little, your eyes will suffer just as the rest of your body does.

Because several visual problems are a direct result of nutritional complications, we should take a deeper look at how various parts of the eyes receive their food supply.

The eyes sit in the eye sockets of the skull, with a padding of fatty tissue surrounding the interior regions. The outer layers of the eyes, which maintain the shape of the eyes, are made up of connective tissue, called sclera. This tissue, and the surrounding extraocular eye muscles, receive their vital supply of oxygen and nutrition directly from the surrounding blood vessels.

However, much of the eye has no direct supply of blood. For obvious optical reasons, the inside of the eye must be clear for light to pass through, so the presence of blood vessels inside the eye would make vision nearly impossible.

So the insides of the eye receive food indirectly, which makes proper circulation even more critical.

If we enter the eye as if we are light on its way to the retina, we first pass through the outer layer of the cornea, called conjunctiva.

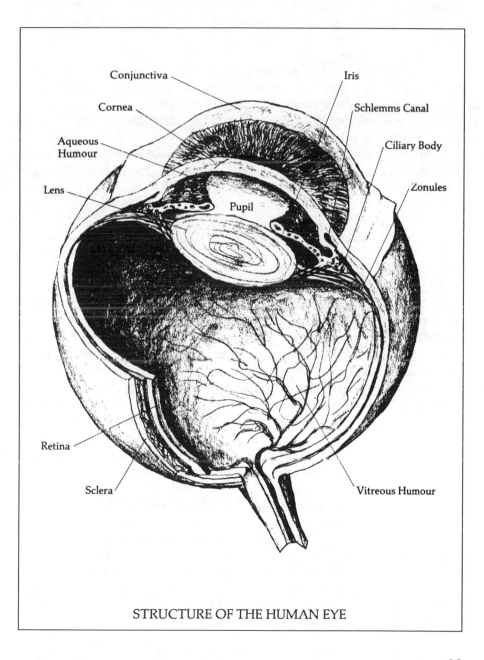

STRUCTURE OF THE HUMAN EYE

Although the surrounding white sclera of the eye has blood vessels, the conjunctiva and cornea do not. They receive their food supply from the liquid directly behind the cornea, called the aqueous humour.

This liquid is constantly being replaced, as its nutrients are depleted, so that every four hours, a complete cycle of circulation of this liquid occurs. The biochemical exchange between the cornea and the aqueous humour is extremely complex, and dependent on factors which scientists still do not fully understand. But adequate nutrition is obviously necessary for the health of the cornea.

As we pass through the aqueous humour, we encounter the inner lens, a marvellous elastic construction which makes our focusing from near to far, and from far to near, possible. The elastic cells which comprise the lens are dependent, like the cells in the cornea, on the aqueous humour for their supply of nutrients and oxygen. There are no blood vessels at all in the lens.

Of vital interest to all of us is that, as we age, the inner cells of the lens often receive inadequate nutrition and begin to die. When this happens, the ability of the lens to change its shape and bend light more strongly, as it must for us to look up close, is reduced. This means that we must resort to reading-glasses as we get older.

But healthy circulation, good diet, and plenty of exercise can logically maintain better circulation in the ocular region, thus keeping the lens cells in better health.

The muscles which control the shape of the lens, called the ciliary muscles, as we mentioned in an earlier chapter, also tend to deteriorate with age, further reducing the up-close focusing ability of the eyes. Both nutrition and visual exercises (the accommodation exercises mentioned before) are important for maintaining healthy ciliary muscles.

Chronic stress in the general musculature of the body generates tension in the ocular muscles as well, and a definite constriction of the circulation. So relaxation is a factor to deal with also with visual health.

To complete our trip to the retina, we leave the lens and move into a relatively large liquid area called the vitreous humour. This liquid, quite unlike the aqueous humour, is not circulated, but is a permanent liquid in the eyes, a type of jelly which serves the function of maintaining the correct shape of the eye. This jelly, like the retina in its back regions, receives its nutrients from the surrounding blood vessels in the sclera.

The retina itself is inlaid with quite a massive network of blood vessels. In fact, a recent innovation in the science of personnel identification uses the unique pattern of blood vessels in the retina as a means of identification.

An irregular or inadequate supply of nutrients to the blood can seriously erode the health of the retina. The retina can even become detached from the back of the eye if nutrition and other factors are disturbed. And of course, the rods and cones themselves, the photosensitive brain cells of the retina, require balanced nutrition for proper functioning.

We now have a complete picture of the inner components of the eyes. The question to be asked at this point is: what about your own physical health? Do your eyes receive proper nutrition from your blood system? Does chronic stress hamper circulation? And do you get enough exercise to maintain optimum circulation of blood to the ocular region?

The following discussion will give you guidelines for evaluation of your condition, and improving that condition if necessary.

There are three principal factors to consider when we look to your health profile. The first is the food you eat, the liquids you drink, and any drugs you take. The second is your exercise routine. The third, often forgotten but vital, is your habital breathing pattern and resultant emotional profile. Each of these factors can be improved without professional help. At this basic level of health, it is your responsibility and your opportunity to take good care of yourself.

First of all, we can consider our eating habits. The general rules of cardio-vascular diet apply also to visual health. Too much intake of animal fat can lead to congestion in the blood vessels, thus reducing circulation. Raw vegetables rich in minerals are always healthy, as are the wholegrain cereals such as rice and wheat. Fruits have their place in a balanced diet, as does protein-rich food such as meat and tofu. To maintain a balanced diet is thus the first pathway to healthy visual functioning.

MOVEMENT

You may have a healthy diet, but the way in which your body processes your food is dependent on your movement habits. Two people can eat the same diet, and yet their bodies can respond to that food intake in quite different ways, depending on their exercise routines. So we turn our focus now to daily routines, to determine whether you might benefit from exercises which directly stimulate circulation and cardio-vascular health.

We have noticed that movement of the eyes is vital for maximum perception. But many of us have habits of not moving the eyes very much, but rather of keeping them locked in staring patterns, inhibiting movement because of various childhood traumas which negatively reinforced active looking.

It is the same with whole-body movement. In fact, the same people who inhibit eye movement often inhibit bodily movement as well.

What about you? Do you like to move? Is it enjoyable to get up and move around, or do you prefer to remain still? Do you regularly exercise enough to get your heart pumping powerfully, so that it remains a dynamic organ, or have you slipped into the habit of low exercise, seldom charging your body with movement and energy?

As with eye habits, it is important not to judge yourself for poor movement habits, but rather to note dispassionately what your present movement profile is and whether it matches your needs for circulatory health.

Many of us have emotional blocks against movement, because such movement does charge our bodies with energy, and we often have habitual blocks against such high levels of energy.

Do you regularly run, dance, jump, play sports, go for vigorous walks, swim, or in other ways charge your body with energy and vitality? Concretely, do you exercise for at least twenty minutes three times a week?

Movement is life. We are constantly in movement, every moment of our lives, from birth to death. Our hearts are beating and our lungs are filling and emptying with air, all the time. Likewise, internal movements of blood are constantly in circulation, lymphatic liquids circulate throughout the body, and the biochemical wonder of our nervous system circulates coded information in constant movement.

To the extent that we freeze our bodies and block the natural tendency to move around, we reduce our vitality, our circulation, and ultimately our visual health as well. There are strong emotional reasons for blocked movement, which we shall explore in the following chapter. For now, we can begin with the basic exercise programme which accompanies this book.

This programme is a unique combination of physical exercise and vision exercise, so that with every whole-body movement that you make, you are also making visual movements. Combined with breathing, this awareness of the eye movement and bodily movement at the same time gives you a dynamic feeling and optimizes the minutes you spend exercising each day.

The third factor in physical/visual health – breathing – reflects the intimate interaction between our physical bodies and our emotional expressions. Each physical movement generates a perfectly matched breathing pattern which balances oxygen needs with carbon dioxide elimination. And each emotional expression also requires a particular breathing pattern. Most movements in fact spring from a mixture of physical and emotional causation.

As a starting point, let's make a simple test. Honestly evaluate your response or reaction right now, as I suggest that you stand up in a moment and do some simple stretching to revitalize your energy level. Do you appreciate this suggestion that you get up and move, after sitting and reading this book, or do you contract away from the suggestion?

- I would love to get up and stretch!
- Oh, maybe it would feel good.
- Actually I feel comfortable.
- What, me exercise? Not a chance.

Of course, our moods change and reflect our interests in movement. But in general, which of the above reactions seems to best express your habits of exercise?

Movement naturally feels good. Our nature is to move. In more primitive conditions, our very survival required regular physical work and movement. Before the advent of the car, we did a great deal more walking. Even riding a horse was good exercise. But now, with such convenient methods of transport, most of us avoid walking when possible.

In addition most human beings in former times did considerable physical work, which stimulated the heart and maintained a healthy cardio-vascular profile. Nowadays we praise modern technology for inventing machines that do most of our physical work for us. The result is that our life-styles demand insufficient exercise to keep us healthy. So we must consciously reverse this pattern, through finding movement programmes which we enjoy and which replace physical work.

I would like to explore with you some movements which generate specific alterations in your breathing, your heart-rate, your perceptual vitality, and your mental alertness. If you cannot stand up and do these exercises right now, it would probably serve you well to return to this part of the discussion again, when you have the time and space to get up and play with the movements.

I use the word 'play' consciously, because if you approach these exercises as 'work', they will not benefit you nearly as much as if you relax, enjoy the movements, and find the pleasure inherent in each exercise. As with eye exercises, whole-body movements should not be forced, but rather should be explored to see what new feelings come from the movements.

We can now progress through the exercise programme. You will find at the end of this section, different arrangements of these exercises, so you can choose a two-minute energizing session, a five-minute revitalization session, a ten-minute conditioning session, and a twenty-minute total exercise session.

You can do these exercises in street clothes, but if you can wear loose clothing and perhaps take off your shoes, the exercises will be more enjoyable.

Often, when beginning a session, you feel lazy and resistant to the idea of movement. Simply trust that within a minute or two of beginning to move, you will shift into the enjoyment which almost always accompanies increased action.

STRETCHING

Simply reach up with one hand towards the ceiling or sky, as shown in the illustration, and then reach with the other hand. Inhale as you stretch, and then allow the following exhalation to be deep, perhaps with a sigh.

Visually, look at the backs of your hands as your stretching continues. Arch your back, shift your weight from one foot to the other, and allow your pelvic region to move also.

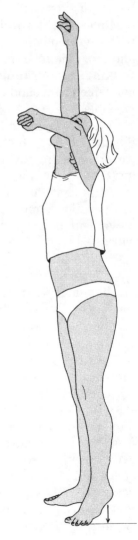

YAWNING

The instinctual stretch of your body is the yawn reflex. This is a natural movement of the body which is stimulated when the carbon dioxide level of the lungs and bloodstream becomes too high. Your breathing needs to expand, and your body needs to increase its charge. Yawning tenses both the face, the breathing system, and then all the muscles in the body as you inhale – and then releases this tension on the deep sigh of the exhalation, generating relaxation along with the increased vitality.

Inhale through the mouth deeply, making a slight yawning sound. Tense the body, drop the jaw wide open, and exhale with the sigh of relaxation. Notice how your eyes are tensed and then relaxed through this yawning. In fact, yawning can be your eyes' best friend.

NECK ROLLS

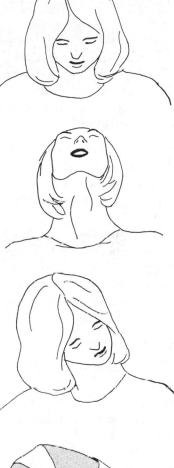

Tension in the neck reflects tension in the ocular region, as numerous studies have documented. So our next step is to move the head around in a slow circle, as shown in the drawing, to relax the neck and shoulder muscles.

Inhale as your head moves upwards in the circle, and exhale as it moves down and forward. Breathe through the mouth, and make a sighing sound for added results.

Visually, let your eyes passively watch the surroundings go by as you make a great circle. The eyes can be out of focus for this, simply relaxing and experiencing the movement. After two or three circles, you can reverse the direction.

It is also fine to do this exercise with the eyes closed, but continuing with the sighing sound of the mouth.

REVERSE-GRAVITY HANG

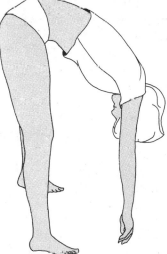

This following exercise is powerful for visual circulation and muscular relaxation in the ocular region. Bend your knees and slowly bend forward and down, with your arms relaxed.

Exhale down with a sigh, until you touch the floor. Remain in this position for a minute, breathe through the mouth, shake the head gently so that the tongue relaxes and the eyes feel the reverse-gravity pull. Then slowly come upright again, breathe deeply, blink regularly.

45

HEAD STIMULATION

Either with open fingers or closed fists, pound gently but firmly on your head. Breathe through the mouth and make a gentle 'aaahh' sound, as you stimulate the circulation of the skull, and especially as you shake the eyes in their orbits, encouraging muscular relaxation.

With your eyes open, experience the shaking of your visual field as you pound all over your head. Especially for the eyes, pound the lower back of the head, where the visual centre of the brain exists. Notice how this also reduces neck tensions.

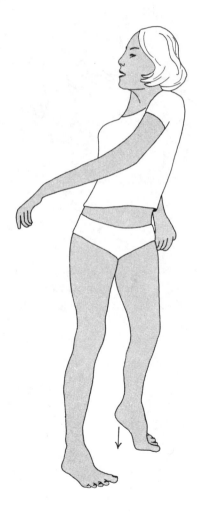

LONG SWINGS

This is a traditional vision-improvement exercise which serves several purposes at once. Stand with your feet fairly wide apart, and slowly turn to look directly behind you, first in one direction, then in the other.

Allow your arms to move with complete relaxation as they naturally swing around your body with the movement. Lift the opposite heel off the floor slightly as you swing, for added pelvic stretching.

Breathe deeply either through the mouth or nose, and blink regularly as you passively watch the environment go by. Let the movement feel enjoyable, natural, relaxed.

FENCER'S STRETCH

One of the innovative exercises for vision and body movement, this is a powerful accommodation exercise for the ciliary muscles, as well as a dynamic breathing routine and a body-coordination movement.

Stand with one foot pointed forward, and the other at right angles to the side, about a foot apart. Clasp your hands together with interlocked fingers behind you, and turn at the waist to look down at one of your feet.

As you *exhale*, bend *both* knees as you bend over the foot you are looking at, so that your head moves towards that bent knee. Keep your knees wide apart, and make sure that you bend your back knee as much as the front one, so that your movement is directly down, not forward.

The vision exercise is to continue to look at the foot throughout three or four cycles of bending over the foot, and then slowly, on the *inhale*, standing up straight again. In this way, your focal distance moves from about one foot directly above your big toe, to the standing distance of about

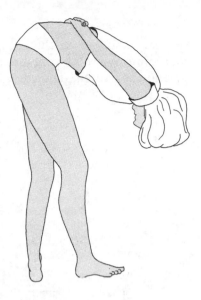

five feet. To match physical movement of this sort with the visual shifting is mysteriously very powerful in activating more dynamic visual habits.

After several cycles over one foot, rotate your position to look down at the opposite foot, and repeat the exercise.

JUMPING/CHARGING

We will now rapidly accelerate the heart-rate and the breathing rate, through gently jumping on one spot. There is a technique for jumping which is especially potent.

Have your feet about a foot apart, or more if you wish. Jump softly, with your feet just coming off the ground. *Inhale* for two jumps, through the mouth, and then exhale for the next two jumps, and maintain this even, fairly slow jumping rhythm.

Make sure your shoulders are relaxed, so that they move up and down with each jump, in accordance with gravity.

Notice how your visual field experiences this jumping. Blink regularly, and allow the bouncing of the outside world to amuse you, with no attempts to focus on any point. Your eyes are once again being shaken in their sockets, encouraging relaxation of the extraocular eye muscles.

Jump till you feel like stopping. Never force yourself to jump beyond the first ten breaths. Your energy level will rise to express your present potential, and to push beyond that is not productive for this programme.

RUNNING

You can also run on the spot, or go jogging, for similar effects. By remaining aware of your breathing and your visual experience, you expand the exercise considerably.

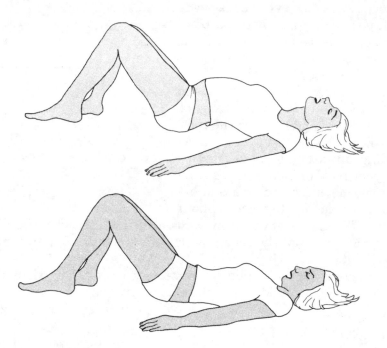

PELVIC ROCK

Lie down on a comfortable rug or other fairly firm surface, with your knees bent and feet flat on the ground. Have your feet and knees about a foot or so apart from each other.

As you *inhale* through the nose, arch your back so that the lower back comes off the floor. Rotate the pelvis back to accompany this natural inhaling movement, and feel the general relaxation which flows throughout the body.

As you *exhale*, through the mouth, reverse the movement. Flatten the lower back against the floor, push with the legs and feet to further this flattening, and rotate the pelvis up and forward assertively.

Exhale completely, contracting the stomach muscles to push all the air out of your lungs. Make a sighing sound of pleasre on the exhale, starting high and finishing with powerful, lusty, low sounds of pushing.

Hold the breath for a moment after the exhalation, to feel your natural hunger for the next inhale. Then, before allowing any air to rush into your lungs, begin to rotate the pelvis and arch the back. After you feel this relaxation in the pelvic region, allow the air to rush into your lungs, effortlessly.

Once you know the movement and breathing pattern, you can focus your attention on your *closed* eyes. Feel the tensing on the exhale, and enjoy the relaxed sensation of the ocular region on the inhale. Make sure that you allow yourself to surrender fully to the pleasure of these movements!

SHOULDER STAND

Taken from the yoga tradition, this posture brings an instant rush of circulation to the ocular region, and allows the eyes and eye muscles to experience an opposite pull of gravity, thus stimulating relaxation and increased eye/brain awareness.

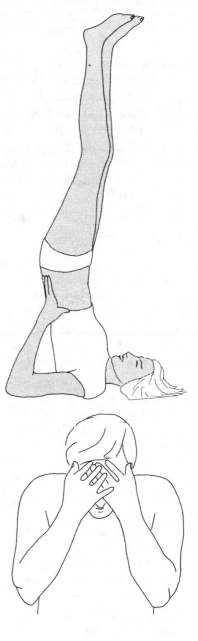

Raise your feet up over your head, using your hands for support under your hips, as shown in the illustration. There is no need for gymnastic perfection here; simply find the general posture which feels good to you.

Breathe evenly through either the nose or the mouth, whichever is more comfortable at the moment. And especially, experience the unique sensations in the eyes! Do this exercise with the eyes closed, except when you strongly prefer eyes open.

PALMING MEDITATION

After lying for a moment following the shoulder stand posture, come to a sitting position and sit cross-legged or on a chair. Cover your eyes in the palming position as learned at the end of Chapter 1, lower your head into your hands so the neck is relaxed, and breathe deeply through either the mouth or the nose for a few cycles. Allow the eyes to relax, and your awareness of your body to expand.

49

5 · VISUAL HEALTH AND EMOTIONAL HEALTH

Perhaps it seems surprising to find a chapter on emotional health in a book about vision. Traditionally, the two subjects have remained in their separate corners, with very little interaction. Visual health was a matter of medicine and optometrics, whereas emotional health was a topic of psychology and psychotherapy.

But a continually expanding understanding of how our emotions affect our bodies has led to a new perception of emotional interaction with the visual system. This discussion will hopefully shed general light on this newly emerging model of emotional/visual integration.

FEAR

Perhaps the clearest starting point is the effect of fear on vision. When we become frightened, our physical vision is reduced. Especially when the fear is prolonged into chronic anxiety, the emotional tendency is towards avoidance of the outside world, which includes the visual world. Fear dilates the pupil, thus reducing visual acuity at the optic level. The breathing is hindered, reducing general circulation and mobility, and the extraocular eye muscles contract and reduce visual movement.

So a person who is generally anxious, with shallow chest breathing and inhibited movement, will also suffer from reduced visual activity. Especially with children in this state, numerous perception habits can develop which reduce visual interaction and perceptual processing.

Conversely, anger which is not mixed with fear has the opposite effect on perception. The pupils contract and thus increase visual acuity. The breathing is powerful and in harmony with bodily movement. The factor of eye mobility is enhanced considerably. And mental alertness is enhanced, increasing the rate of visual processing and association.

We will leave for later chapters the explanation of how fear affects conditions such as myopia, glaucoma, and eye allergies. This chapter will deal with the more universal condition of stress and tension, which leads to eye aches, headaches, shoulder tension, and general inhibition of the visual system.

Stress is a physiological condition. It occurs when the body responds to a perceived danger with the physical condition called 'arousal'. First there is a reaction of fear, which is a powerful inhalation and then a discharge of the energy generated by the fear reaction. In arousal, fear is the first part of a general response of action, of assertion to deal successfully with the danger.

But in a stress situation, there is no immediate physical reaction which will eliminate the danger. So the body charges itself for action, but has no means of discharging the excited state in assertion. Tension therefore exists in the body. And this tension exists in the eyes as well as throughout the muscular system of the body in general. Is this a condition you experience personally?

The modern world is full of threats which generate the arousal response inside us, but which allow for no physical discharge and resolution. For example, the constant threat of the nuclear bomb naturally threatens us and evokes the arousal response, especially with children. But there is nothing we can do to act against the danger. We cannot attack and eliminate the threat. We cannot run away from it. So we are caught in a stressful situation.

In primitive times, where our arousal reactions were developed as instinctual patterns, a direct danger could be dealt with through direct fighting or running away. But in contemporary business and social life, we suppress our overt emotions, controlling our instinctual responses through learned inhibition.

This inhibition helps a complex society such as ours function successfully. But it also takes its toll on the body. Stress is a symptom which generates heart complications, high blood-pressure, chronic anxiety and tensions, ulcers, backaches and headaches, mental confusion – and visual disorders as well.

If you are faced with a danger which you cannot eliminate through attacking or running away, your only remaining choice is to ignore the danger and pretend that it doesn't exist. This is the source of many habitual perception patterns which directly reduce our ability to see the outside world. And because we develop these habits mostly unconsciously, we are not aware that we are even hindering our vision. Most people with such perceptual blocks don't know they have them.

But once you read a discussion such as this, and become alerted to such unconscious patterns, you can begin to reverse the old habits. Once you see what you are doing to yourself, a natural correction begins to take place, overriding the outdated habit with new, realistic habits.

It is curious that the state of anxiety, of chronic arousal, has just the opposite effect in short-term situations to the one it is meant to have. When we are held in the state of arousal with no relief, our ability to survive is actually reduced. If we cannot act and reduce our charge of energy in the body, we find ourselves locked in tensions and perceptual inhibitions that get in our way.

So as a general visual health programme, we need to explore several concrete exercises which will enable us to overcome habitual states of anxiety and stress. To do this, we first turn to the breathing, because this primary act of respiration is inhibited by stress, and must be corrected if we are to promote general relaxation throughout the body.

If anxiety and stress are blocked expressions of assertion at the physical level, the resolution of the condition is to move in such ways as to discharge the tensions. Assertion is also a visual experience; we can see the brightness in a person's eyes when there is a freedom of expression. So we can encourage this feeling in the eyes as well as in the body. Try the following exercise and notice its effects.

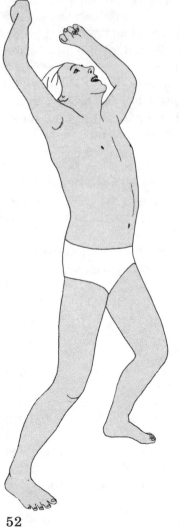

PERSONAL POWER

Stand up with your feet fairly wide apart. As you *inhale*, raise your arms up over your head, with your hands powerfully clenched. Inhale deeply as you arch your back and feel the power implied in this gesture.

Especially, feel the altered energy level in your eyes as you play with this posture of assertion. You will notice that the feeling of power and pressure in your body in general is also felt in the eyes.

Now, as you begin to *exhale* through the mouth, bring your arms forward and down, as if to hit a table in front of you at waist-height. Bend your knees as you swing your arms down, so that your torso remains *upright*, not bent forward.

At first, make this movement gently, playfully, saying 'Haaaiiiii-yaaahhhh!' as you exhale and bring your arms down. Then bring your arms up again with the next *inhale*, fully charging your body. Hold that inhalation a moment as you start the 'Haaaaaiiiiii' sound, and then as you slowly but powerfully swing your arms and fists forward and down, discharge the pressure in your chest with the 'Yaaahhhhhh' sound of hitting.

Notice the increase in energy which you feel as you do this perhaps six times, increasing your speed and power with each cycle. Be sure to continue smiling as you do this exercise, to keep the energy light and expansive.

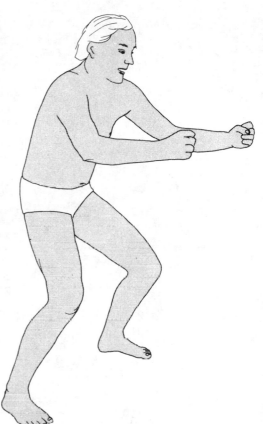

Visual vitality is a quality which we all know exists, because we can see it in other people's eyes. Science is still trying to pinpoint the electro-chemical dimensions of visual vitality, but regardless of the scientific confusion right now regarding its origin, the relative liveliness or emptiness of a person's eyes is a phenomenon we can work with to increase.

Medicine is currently caught in a quandary regarding the proper model for the physical body. Practical results of such non-Western medical techniques as acupuncture indicate that there is indeed a level of energy flow in the body which we cannot fully comprehend at the present.

The same is true with the psychological traditions of such doctors as Wilhelm Reich and Alexander Lowen, who have explored the flow of excitation through the body related to emotional discharge.

With regards to vision, certain emotional blocks also cause a blockage of excitation in the ocular region of the body. This means that the general vitality of the eyes is reduced, due to emotional inhibition. Childhood punishment for being assertive, angry, and resistant tends to lead to this ocular blocking.

We can leave the scientists to explain more fully the biochemical dynamics of ocular vitality, and move on to the practical exercises which stimulate this energy flow in the eyes.

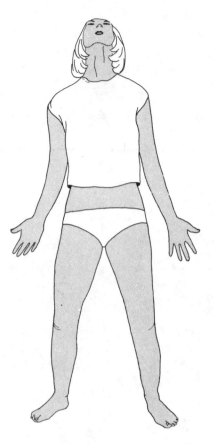

FEAR/ASSERTION

This exercise directly stimulates the visual expression of vitality and assertiveness, breaking through old inhibitions through conscious movement. Give the exercise a try to find out how your own eyes respond to this type of rejuvenation.

Stand with your feet fairly wide apart, and first of all, on the *inhale*, imitate the posture of fear in the body. Imagine that something has suddenly surprised you, and you inhale sharply in shock, straighten your knees, arch your back, and look upwards in the classic shock posture, as shown in the illustration.

Now that you have this charge of energy in your body, the result of the fear response, *exhale* powerfully to discharge that energy, jumping onto your feet with the knees bent and the hands on the knees, your vocal expression making a growling sound of power and your eyes expressing this feeling also.

Then on the *inhale*, return to the fear, charging posture, your arms back and your head up, inhaling deeply. And discharge that new excitation through jumping onto your crouched legs again, feeling your expression flowing out through your eyes. Do this in front of a mirror, or facing a friend who is also doing the exercise at the same time, so further explore this release of visual power and vitality.

Repeat the cycle four or five times.

Notice that you can do this exercise with an angry hardness as your feeling, or with an enjoyable sense of power mixed with the pleasure of

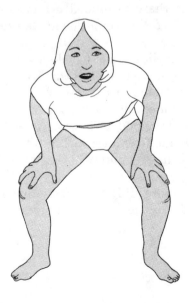

assertion. My personal preference with this type of exercise is to include a smile on the face, to encourage the positive association of assertion (anger in the extreme) with pleasure (satisfaction of emotional expression).

A more subtle approach to this factor of energy levels in the eyes is to deal with the habitual expressions which we hold on our faces. Most of us spend most of our waking hours either smiling automatically to be socially friendly, or going around with a controlled, stern expression on our faces. Take a look around you as you walk down a street or sit on a bus: few people have relaxed faces. This chronic tension of the facial muscles directly affects the tension in the ocular muscles, and therefore should be concretely dealt with.

The following exercise is most helpful.

THE INNER SMILE

Rather than tensing the face for a full social smile, relax the facial muscles completely, letting your jaw drop slightly open so that the tongue and jaw muscles are also relaxed.

Now imagine that there is a slight inner smile beginning to radiate deep within you. This inner smile includes a feeling of energy flowing towards the eyes, as opposed to the downward-flowing sensation of a forced smile.

Breathe into this upward-flowing sensation, and allow it to reach the eyes and invigorate them as well.

We can now advance a further step in the vision/emotions dimension.

After reading this description of the exercise, shut your eyes and imagine something which currently bothers you in life, threatens you somehow, scares you even. This can be a person, a situation – whatever. Just allow this threat to grow in your inner eye.

FACING YOUR DANGER

The purpose of this exercise is to turn and look directly at something which you are afraid of, and therefore tend to avoid facing.

The act of avoiding something which threatens you is a natural reaction of fear. But in most cases, it is not a positive reaction for survival these days. Unfortunately, we have childhood habits which conditioned us to avoid looking at anything which scared or repulsed us.

Now you can directly act to reverse that habit of visual avoidance. Imagine that you are turning and are now directly looking at something which you usually avoid facing. Notice what happens.

What happens to your breathing for instance?

This is an exercise to do many times, as are most of the others. You need to explore your habits repeatedly, allowing them to shift and to outgrow old contractions. Notice that if you concentrate on your exhale, on that feeling of the fear/assertion exercise, you will have more success in visualizing this confrontation with your dangers in life. And when you face your dangers, they almost always appear less dangerous!

6 · RELAXATION

We have seen in the previous chapter that active exercises can reduce stress considerably. This present chapter shows the other approach to stress reduction – direct focusing on relaxation.

We should take the stretching/yawning reflex as our ideal model of natural relaxation. First, the body tenses and further contracts the muscles. Then comes the relaxation stage. In like manner, you should do the fear/assertion exercise if you are tense, before beginning with these relaxation exercises.

For most of us, our extraocular muscles surrounding the eyes, and the ciliary muscles inside the eyes, are overly tense. If we could only directly massage these muscles, there would be a simple method for dealing with this chronic tension. But the muscles are unavailable for direct contact. So we must turn to the next most practical methods of relaxation.

First begin with the whole body. If the muscles of your body in general receive orders from the brain to relax, you can be certain that the visual muscles receive relaxation suggestions also.

Relaxation is a natural response of the body following physical exertion. What we want to do is to activate this natural process. So first do some jumping, or the personal power exercise, or the fear/assertion movements. Breathe powerfully and allow your body to develop a sense of increased vitality. Notice how these exercises are affecting your eyes.

Then, to further stimulate the ocular muscles, do the head stimulation exercise, pounding on your head to shake the eyes and loosen the surrounding muscles. The reverse-gravity hang will also help in this first step towards visual relaxation and tension reduction.

WHOLE BODY RELAXATION

Find a comfortable place where you can lie quietly for perhaps five to ten minutes. Be sure you will be warm and undisturbed. Perhaps take the phone off the hook, and lock your door if you need that sense of complete security.

Lie on your back with your knees bent and feet on the ground, and do the pelvic rock exercise you have already learned. Tense your whole body on the exhale, further stimulating all the muscles in your body. Then, on the inhale, sense the spontaneous inflow of fresh air as you relax and allow the breathing process to occur.

Now allow your legs to lie flat on the ground, with a small pillow under the knees if this is more comfortable. With your eyes closed, turn your focus completely to your breathing and discover what happens when you make absolutely no effort to breathe. Let your breath stop after your next exhale, and see if there is a natural inner force which will bring about your next inhale, without you making any conscious effort.

Continue to watch your breathing, feeling the location in your body where your inhale seems to begin. Go through perhaps ten breath cycles, as you relax step by step.

TENSION/RELAXATION EXERCISE

Continuing in the same position on the floor, inhale and tense the muscles in your feet a moment. Then as you exhale, relax your feet, and feel how this tensing/relaxing process generates deeper relaxation.

Now tense your legs as you inhale, then relax them as you exhale. You can do this with one leg at a time if you want, or both together. After a tensing cycle, breathe for one breath cycle before going further, to allow a conscious awareness of the progressive relaxation.

The third step in this relaxation is to tense your buttock muscles as you inhale (your legs and feet will probably also tense and this is fine) and then relax completely as you exhale. Breathe through another cycle and observe how you are more fully relaxed now.

As you inhale for the fourth step, arch your back and tense your spine, chest, and arms together. Hold this tension a moment on the full inhale, and then exhale and relax.

For the fifth step, arch your neck and tense your neck and facial muscles on the inhale, and then relax as you exhale.

Finally, tense your entire body at once, from feet to fists to head, as you inhale. Then sigh through the mouth as you exhale, and allow all the remaining tensions to flow out of you. Let your next inhale be effortless, and continue breathing as complete relaxation fills your body!

EYE MASSAGE

Another technique for a visual relaxation is drawn from the Chinese acupressure tradition, employing the fingers to provide stimulation to points which are related with visual relaxation.

Either sitting or lying down, place your thumbs over your temples and arch your fingers so that the forefingers are over the eyebrows. Begin with the fingers touching each other. As you slowly exhale, pull the forefingers across the eyebrows, pressing firmly as you do so, thus stimulating the four acupressure points which lie along this line of the eyebrows. You will probably notice the points as you move over them.

Inhale as you move your fingers back to the first position, and then repeat this movement three or four times, always on the exhale. Then cover your eyes with your hands in the palming position (see end of Chapter 1) and relax further.

GUIDED RELAXATION SESSION

We now advance to a deeper level of relaxation. This technique, employed professionally for visual relaxation and recovery, is related to hypnosis, but should not be confused with classic hypnosis. There will be no hypnotic post-condition suggestion included in these sessions. We are simply going to go on a guided journey into the regions of our inner selves where communication between the brain and the eyes occurs.

You can either read through this session, remember the steps, and go through them yourself, or you can make a simple tape-recording for yourself as a guide.

Lie down comfortably on your back, and bring your focus to your breathing. With every inhalation, fill yourself with peace and relaxation, and with every exhalation, allow the tensions in your mind and body to flow out of you and be gone. Spend perhaps ten breath cycles on this beginning step, as you move deeper into a state of quiet, calm relaxation.

Bring your focus to the actual air rushing in and out your nose, and feel the sensation of the stimulation occurring inside your nose.

Allow this awareness to expand so that you are aware of your whole head at once, of the volume inside your skull. With every inhalation, allow this awareness to expand, until you feel deeply conscious of your own brain.

From this deep level of awareness, allow your attention to expand another step, to include awareness of your eyes themselves. Don't make any effort to do this, and don't play mind games about what this awareness would be like. Simply see directly what genuine awareness you can have of your eyes, when you are also aware of breathing through your nose, and of your brain itself.

Notice without judgement the level of tension in your eyes. Accept how you are right now, breathe into your present level of tension or relaxation, watching with interest to see what happens next.

With the next inhalation, say to yourself the word 'relax'. With your next exhalation, repeat the word 'relax'. Hold your focus on your eyes, so that the mental suggestion is directed to this region of your body.

Continue with this verbal suggestion for perhaps ten breath cycles, feeling the expression of the word subliminally on your tongue, and allowing your throat to relax also.

Expand this sense of relaxation, with every inhalation and exhalation, so that your facial muscles relax step by step too. Notice how intimately related the facial muscles are to the extraocular eye muscles.

Now just relax and notice how your eyes feel. Let your awareness expand to include all of your body at once, in an effortless expansion of consciousness that requires no cognitive activity at all. Just breathe and be aware of your body on the floor, from head to toes at once.

FACIAL RELAXATION

To relax the face further, at any time of the day, there is a four-breath exercise which is extremely powerful and pleasurable.

Place your hands over your face, with the palms over your eyes and your fingers above your forehead, as shown. Inhale deeply, and then as you *exhale*, bring your fingers down over your face very slowly. Have the fingers arched slightly, so that your fingertips move slowly over your face.

Sigh through the mouth as you do this, and feel how your fingers seem to relax the facial muscles as they pass over them, taking any remaining tension away.

Let your fingers continue down over your chin and down your neck, removing tension from that region. Then make a quick shake of the fingers, as if throwing away the tension gathered from the face.

Do this four times, on the exhale, and then simply relax with the hands over the eyes in the palming position. Your face and eyes should be significantly more relaxed now, your breathing deep and rhythmic, and you body enjoyably relaxed as well.

BREATHING THROUGH THE EYES

This final exercise in this relaxation chapter combines breathing, awareness of your actual eyes, and the mental imagery of breathing through the eyes as well as the nose. The results, as you will find, are quite dramatic, providing perhaps the most effective means for relaxing the extraocular eye muscles, and the ciliary muscles as well.

First with the eyes closed, be aware of the air as it rushes in and out through your nose for a few cycles, as you relax and move into a deeper awareness of your body.

Now imagine that the air is also flowing in through your eyes in the *inhale*, and out through your eyes on the *exhale*. Allow your jaw muscle to relax, your tongue to relax, and your eyes to relax.

With every inhalation, imagine that you are bringing healing love and relaxation into your eyes, and with every exhalation, imagine that you are sending your own vitality and presence out into the world. Feel as if energy is flowing into you through your eyes, and then out through your eyes.

Notice that there is an actual physical shifting which occurs in the eyes as you visualise this 'breathing through the eyes' experience. The eyes move slightly back as you inhale, and then relax and move slightly forward as you exhale. This actual movement is remarkably effective in reducing visual tension, and in enhancing eye/brain harmony and communication.

Continue with this breathing for as long as you want!

7 · LIGHT, LIGHTING, AND EYE-STRAIN REDUCTION

Obviously, without an initial light source in the environment, we would have no visual experience at all. The visual perception of the outside world is totally dependent on light.

Light itself is a form of radiant energy, coming either from the natural sources such as the sun, fires, lightning, etc., or from man-made sources such as electrically fired lightbulbs and discharge lamps (sodium and phosphorus-coated fluorescent lamps).

Light is basically a very small part of the electromagnetic spectrum which itself ranges from the extremely rapid wavelengths of cosmic rays, to the very slow wavelengths of radio waves. Visible light is a frequency range of radiation which is absorbed by the photo-receptors of the retina, thus beginning the process of seeing.

LIGHT AND THE VISUAL SYSTEM

Our eyes function at different levels of performance, depending partly on the type of lighting which is available for the visual work. When the lighting is optimal, we see very clearly, have very little eye-strain, and can process visual information quite quickly. The converse is true if the lighting is poor.

So we should ask the question, what in fact are the qualities of 'good lighting'? First of all, the light must be bright enough so that the photo-receptors of the retina are adequately stimulated. Otherwise, the interpreting part of the brain must work over-hard to guess what is actually being seen. This guessing generates mental fatigue.

If lighting is dim, people also have a natural tendency to get closer to the visual task, thus increasing the work of the ciliary muscles in close-up accommodation, and also making the extraocular muscles work harder because the eyes must converge more when an object is closer to them.

Although there will be no direct damage to the eyes if you read by candlelight, for instance, for a reasonable amount of time, you will generate eye-strain through the above-mentioned complications.

Another factor in lighting is glare, of reflection from surfaces of a bright, distracting light which interferes with visual processing. Glare generates muscle tensions in the eyebrows and face as well, leading to possible headaches.

SUNLIGHT AND HEALTH

Indirect sunlight is one of the best sources of light for the human eye, and when possible, reading or other visual tasks should be done by sunlight. But when there is direct sunlight, the glare factor develops conditions leading to eye-strain and mental fatigue.

One quality of sunlight which is lost with artificial lighting is the constant variety of intensity and shadow of sunlight, as the earth spins through its daily cycle from night to day and into darkness again. This constantly changing source of light from the sun allows the eyes to function in different ways at different luminations and angles of light, thus keeping the visual system fresh and relaxed. When lighting is fixed, the eyes become more rigid in their performance, and eye-strain can result, along with a reduction in visual processing.

It is very unfortunate that so many of our modern school buildings have been built with very little glass to permit natural lighting while children are indoors doing schoolwork, and architects designing new schools should bear this in mind. Artificial lighting should only be necessary through reduced sunlight in winter, during cloudy days, and at night.

Although still the subject of controversy, it has been demonstrated that for the optimum health the human body needs periodic inputs of the full spectrum of natural radiant light, as various glands are affected by this input. Without it, general health can be eroded.

This energy enters through the eyes, and also through the surface of the skin, penetrating deeply into the body with healthful vibratory stimulation. Both for adults working inside buildings every day, and for children in school and at home, serious consideration should be given to regular exposure to sunlight. Even when it is cloudy, by the way, this healthy stimulation occurs.

At deep levels, our bodies seem to run in cyclic harmony with the rotation of the earth, and the night–day cycles. To lose touch with these primary earthly cycles, through not coming into contact with the constantly changing angles of sunlight from night to day, and through the four seasons, appears to be detrimental to our health.

It is curious that many people do not even know in which direction our planet is spinning through space. We are in fact sitting on a tiny ball speeding through blank space, linked with our sun as the primary reference point in the universe, day in and day out. Primitive people were very conscious of the position of the sun, could tell time very closely by just glancing at its position in the sky, and maintained an intimate relationship with sunlight.

But with the introduction of artificial light, mostly since the turn of the century, we have become independent of sunlight for our visual tasks, and thus have lost much contact with our orientation regarding sun position. For instance, can you point right now in the direction in which our planet is spinning through space?

Through logic, we can quickly realize that we must be spinning east, because that is the direction the sun appears to rise from. So if we sit facing east, we are facing 'forward' on the planet, and if we sit facing west, we are facing 'backwards'. A simple meditation on this direction and sense of movement of the planet every day, just for a few minutes, perhaps while watching the sun rise or set, will give you an immediately deeper contact with this amazing world we are blessed to live upon.

In traditional times, many cultures worshipped the sun. Certainly this natural response to the provider of the energy which makes life possible on the planet should continue to reverberate through our systems, if we open ourselves to the simple realities of planetary life.

PROPER LIGHTING FOR EASE OF SEEING

In general, when doing close-up work, lighting should be over the shoulder so that there is no direct glare of light into the eyes. Also, the light should strike the surface being looked at (such as the page of a book) with an oblique angle rather than a right angle, so that there is not a direct reflection of glare back into the eyes.

Parents are often too strict and too worried about the reading and lighting habits of children. We should keep in mind that although temporary eye-strain might result from glare and dim lighting, permanent damage almost never occurs. The exceptions are with infra-red light, direct looking at the sun, etc., where tissue damage is possible. Looking directly into the sun with the eyes open is very dangerous and can create permanent retinal damage.

Comfort is the general rule for lighting. You want to see what you are looking at clearly, without muscle tension, with intensity of light matching the visual situation. Psychologists and light specialists are working with complex ways of measuring productivity related to lighting, and this is certainly an interesting study, making the work we do more comfortable visually. But common sense can usually tell you how best to light your homes and office space.

Fluorescent lights are still a matter of controversy. In past days, many schools used light bulbs which did not emit the full spectrum of visible light, thus depriving children and adults of vital electromagnetic stimulation. But this situation can be corrected through the use of full-spectrum lamps. You should check in your home, office, and schools to make sure that full-spectrum lamps are in fact being used.

There has also been considerable controversy over the effect of the high-speed flicker of many fluorescent lamps. In fact, certain rates of flicker can harm the functioning of the mind, and in extreme cases can cause some people to suffer from epileptic fits and hyperactivity. Once again, the functioning of fluorescent lamps has been greatly improved recently, and it appears that this flicker problem is not now a serious factor in properly functioning lamp units.

In general, the more aware we are of factors such as glare and intensity of light, the more successfully we will adjust our various light sources to provide maximum comfort in visual activities. There is always an optimum balance between distance from a light source, and intensity of the light source. Finding your favourite balance is one of the creative aspects of daily life. The more conscious we are of our lighting habits, the more freedom of adjustment and choice we will find.

REDUCING EYE-STRAIN

Certainly the most effective way to treat eye-strain is to close the eyes and do the palming exercise already introduced. This exercise provides maximum opportunity both for relaxing the ocular muscles, and for relieving the brain of perceptual work for a short time.

Nearly all visual tasks, except those like driving a car, provide space for you to pause and palm for a few moments. Remember that through combining awareness of your breathing with the palming relaxation exercise, you exponentially enhance the effects of palming, because by doing so you also relax the tensions in your breathing mechanism which are a primary source of tension throughout the body.

Another principle eye-strain-reduction exercise is simple jumping, or any movement which frees the eyes and breaks fixated visual patterns. Neck rolls are excellent for reducing eye-strain as well. And the accommodation exercise of holding a finger close to your eyes, and then shifting your focus into the distance, serves to relax the ocular muscles which must work very hard to focus up-close over a period of time.

Regular pauses to look into the distance, in fact, are a primary eye-strain prevention exercise. If you stop working the eyes at a particular task and allow them to feel free for a few moments just to look around where they please, you are tapping both the physiological and the emotional path to eye-strain reduction. To the extent that the eyes are treated like slaves that must perform constantly under stress, there will be eye-strain. To the extent that the eyes feel free for part of each hour, they will function with minimum tensions.

And finally, even when you are reading or doing some up-close visual task, you can remain aware of your breathing, and see how your habits of holding your breath and not exhaling completely lead towards eye-strain conditions. Conscious awareness of the breathing will spontaneously improve the breathing!

8 · COMMON VISUAL DIFFICULTIES

TELEVISION

During the last fifty years the advent of the television and the computer terminal has brought about a drastic alteration in most of our daily visual activities. What are the effects of television and computer terminal watching?

Children watch television many hours a day, almost every day of their lives. Instead of being outside, playing games which involve varied ocular activity, children spend many hours with their eyes fixed on a relatively small, unmoving area of the potential visual field.

This means that the extraocular eye muscles, which control the direction the eyes look, must maintain a relatively static, tense posture, for relatively long periods of time. The closer to the television a child sits, the more extraocular strain there will be, as the eyes must converge more strongly when looking up-close.

Thus, a general rule would indicate that getting back away from the television, at least five feet, is a healthy practice, reducing eye-strain.

Controversy still continues about the different physiological effects of chronic television viewing. The cathode-ray tube definitely shoots rays out into your eyes, rays which do not occur naturally in such intensities but which we are suddenly exposing entire generations to. The radiation emission of television sets has been reduced noticeably, but it is certainly still present. And the closer you sit, the more intense the radiation.

Head posture in viewing television for a period of time should also be considered. Many children maintain stress postures while watching television, mainly for emotional reasons beyond the scope of this discussion. Bringing to consciousness these habitual bodily contortions can, in itself, generate a natural correction.

But once again, no serious damage has been noticed from abnormal head positions, and aside from occasional eye-strain, people seldom complain about the detrimental visual effects of television viewing. Obviously, the longer you force your eyes to perform the very rigid task of watching a television screen, the more deleterious the visual effects will be.

Notice, for example, that when you sit watching television, your ciliary muscles, which control focusing in the eyes, must maintain a constant, unchanging muscle tension. We all know that muscles become fatigued faster when held in one stress position, than when allowed to move freely in a wide range of movements. The same is true for the eyes.

So when you or your children watch television, remember that the eyes will love you if you simply look off into the distance with every commercial or station break. Give the muscles a chance to relax!

Certainly, breath awareness is vital in watching television too, especially because suspense dramas and the like tend to freeze the diaphragm muscle with the fear response.

COMPUTERS AND THE EYES

The same basic logic applies both to television and video display units. The closer you are to the screen, the more extraocular and ciliary tension you will develop. The more you stare at the screen, the more rigid and fatigued the eyes will become. And the longer you look at a fixed distance, the more tension you generate in the accommodation muscles.

Great advances have been made in the actual numbers and letters printed on the VDU. In less recent times, the presentation of material on the screen was often blurry, poorly illuminated, and prone to a jumpy quality which generated rapid visual and mental fatigue.

Recent VDU improvements, such as employing soothing, glare-reducing colours for background, and establishing proper contrast between foreground and background, have helped computer operators considerably. Progress is still being made in this field.

But in general, we should remember that our eyes were not naturally designed for such work at all, and to whatever extent we tax our visual systems with unnatural work, we should compensate with exercises and break periods.

Breathing is another crucial variable. People tend to hold their breath when operating a computer. This generates reduced mental performance and muscular functioning, and is perhaps the most serious complication of regular work at a computer terminal. Conscious awareness of breathing habits will help reduce this problem.

COMPUTER EXERCISES

Getting up and moving your whole body is perhaps the most important regular exercise at the VDU. Stretching, yawning, hanging your head forward and down, breathing through the mouth, jumping, and doing long swings, all of which have been presented before, will help your body recover from periods of taxing visual and mental work.

And developing the simple habit of looking away from the terminal into the distance once every ten minutes is an ideal pattern for reducing eye-strain and mental fatigue.

Palming is another primary exercise, instantly freeing the eyes from their normal work, and also eliminating any visual inputs to the mind, so that a quietness can develop. By watching your breathing while palming, you generate a meditative state which can directly counteract the routine of the computer.

NIGHT DRIVING AND NIGHT BLINDNESS

Driving a car is extremely demanding visual work, even in the daytime. At night, when lighting is greatly reduced and the eyes must shift from cone perception to rod perception, visual performance is still more difficult.

Proper driving requires continual rapid eye movements to scan for moving vehicles, pedestrians, red lights, and all the rest. In fact, driving is a good visual exercise, keeping the eyes active, flexible, quick, and sharp.

There are two primary complications which occur visually when driving. First of all, the routine work of driving for longer than an hour or so can lead to general tiredness and boredom. This loss in mental functioning is directly reflected in perceptual processing of visual data. In fact, a recent study of road accidents showed that 44 per cent of all accidents involved a perceptual error. Of this 44 per cent, 17 per cent of accidents were caused by 'looking but failing to see' errors.

Obviously, if we look at something, but fail to see it, the problem is a function of mental alertness and awareness, not of simple ocular functioning. Mental fatigue can be generated, however, by repetitive visual inputs which tend to hypnotize the driver.

The second complication in driving has to do with the availability of light, and with such factors as glare. These aspects make the basic act of seeing more difficult, regardless of visual and mental alertness.

Night driving generates a special complication because periods of darkness are interspersed with a sudden glaring light from headlamps. The iris which enlarges the pupil for night seeing, must suddenly contract when bright lights appear. Then, following the bright lights of a passing car, the iris must adjust again, a process which takes several minutes in most cases.

So, through an unnatural rapid shifting from bright to dark, the visual functioning of the eyes is reduced, making perception for driving a difficult task, at best.

What can be done to maximize vision for night driving? First of all, for general alertness, we once again return to the factor of breathing. When you become tired while driving, your breathing rate and depth is reduced dramatically. Less oxygen is therefore available for your functioning, and you are not optimally conscious.

A powerful trick for stimulating alert breathing is to exhale strongly through the mouth, making a round 'aaahhhh' sound until you have contracted your abdomen muscles and pushed every bit of air out of your lungs. Then if you hold your breath for a few seconds, you will stimulate your instinctual inhalation reflex, thus bringing your body more into the present.

Also, when you see headlights coming at you in the distance, you can turn your head slightly away from the glare, and blink a little more slowly than usual so that your eyes do not have to react to a constant glaring light source.

Night blindness is usually a genetic complication, where there are no or insufficient rods to process the low levels of incoming light normally dealt with for night vision. There is no known 'cure' for this condition. If you don't have the rods in the retina in the first place, you cannot use this mode of seeing at all.

However, many people have temporary night blindness, caused by constriction of the iris following a sudden exposure to bright lights. For this condition, a few moments suffice for normal vision to be regained.

MINOR EYE-INJURY TREATMENT

Certainly the most common eye injury is a scratching of the surface of the cornea (the epithelium) by a blow to the eye, or an object which enters the eye from the atmosphere. We have all at some time had dust particles in our eyes, usually finding that they are quickly flushed out by the simple action of the tear glands. Many such irritants need no treatment at all, except for allowing a few minutes for the increased tear flow to carry them away.

Slightly more serious, most of us have had the surface of an eye scratched with a fingernail, an unseen branch, or some other sharp object. The cornea is remarkably resilient, and it recovers from slight abrasions very rapidly. If the exterior surface has been scratched away, instant healing begins to take place to replace the damaged or lost cells and return the outer surface of the eye to a normal healthy state. So a minor scratch often does not even require medical treatment, unless the pain is acute.

However, the healing process can be augmented, especially if the pain persists for several hours, through local administration of a painkiller, antibiotics to prevent infection, drops to rest the focusing system of the eye, and a patch to prevent the lid from constantly rubbing against the injured part of the cornea with each blinking action of the eye. Usually minor abrasions will heal in 24 to 48 hours, with or without medical intervention.

A more serious condition occurs when a foreign body, usually a splinter of glass or a metal filing, becomes lodged in the corneal surface. Often these particles are too small even to be seen by the naked eye, and the only way you know there is something in the eye is that every time you blink or move it in the socket a new scratch is generated.

A doctor can very easily do what you simply cannot do at home, in this case. He or she will apply local anaesthetic drops, and then look under a microscope to locate the particle, and then remove it with tiny tweezers. Since there has usually been a break in the surface of the eyeball, applying antibiotics is more crucial here than with simple abrasions. An eye patch will usually be recommended for a couple of days until healing is complete.

All other injuries, such as serious blows to the eye, internal bleeding of the eye, and deeper lacerations of the corneal surface or the eyelid, should be treated professionally as soon as possible.

Perhaps the most important point in this section is to recommend wearing safety glasses in hazardous situations. They are a little awkward, but they can save your vision!

Chemical burns are a special type of eye injury. Immediate irrigation of the eye, flushing it continuously with water, is the first step, before rushing to an emergency ward for treatment by a doctor.

HELP FOR DRY, BURNING, IRRITATED EYES

For eye irritations caused by over-work, smoking, hay fever and allergy complications, and general dry eyes, I recommend a product made from the leaves of the Aloe Vera plant, a plant which is widely known for its healing, soothing qualities. There are several companies which produce such eyedrops from Aloe Vera. You can check with your pharmacist or a health foods store to see which might be in stock. Naturally, if you are having chronic problems with eye irritation, you might want to see a doctor, but in general they will prescribe stronger drops, which in my experience are less effective or not effective at all. Many of the eye doctors these days, however, will recommend Aloe Vera as well.

OUTDOOR SPORTS AND THE EYES

Ever since their introduction into general population use through the image-makers of Hollywood, sunglasses have had a controversial history. Some optometrists recommended wearing sun-glasses whenever in the sun, to reduce eye-strain caused by squinting. Other doctors warned against using sun-glasses, except in extreme glare situations, because wearing them can reduce the normal reaction of the iris and thus debilitate the natural protection against glare, through disuse of the contraction potential of the iris.

A happy medium seems best. It is true that many people become dependent, at least for a period of time, on their sun-glasses, and can't even leave the house without having them in place on sunny days. Other people avoid wearing them altogether, and suffer from eye-strain, headaches, and burning eyes through over-exposure to the glare of snow and sand.

Such sports as skiing obviously dictate sun-glasses. Playing baseball or tennis in the bright sunlight also seems to dictate sun-glasses in most cases. Driving into the sun is difficult – and therefore more dangerous – without sun-glasses. Other than in such extreme conditions, you are probably better off letting your eyes do their own adjusting to sunlight. And wearing a hat in the sun is the traditional means of dealing with glare.

9 · ENHANCING THE PLEASURE OF SEEING

In traditional textbooks, when talking about the act of seeing, authors usually refer to 'performing visual tasks'. Seeing is considered to be work. The eyes are regarded primarily as organs for gathering visual information for one specific purpose or another.

Certainly this is one dimension of seeing. But in this chapter, we are going to explore the opposite side of perception — the simple pleasure of looking at something. Our perceptual habits will dictate, moment to moment, how we are using our eyes. Some of us have such strong habits of working constantly, that we never, or very seldom, pause to enjoy the sensation of perception for its own sake.

VISUAL FREEDOM

As babies and little children, before we were sent to school, we actually spent a great deal of our time looking, purely for the fun of it. We were gathering useful information in the process, but if you follow a small child around for an hour or so, when it is free to do as it wishes, much of its time will be spent in the enjoyment of seeing.

It seems to be a natural function of the human being, this pleasure function. And just as we can enjoy the taste of an orange, we can enjoy looking at a sunset, and can find it equally satisfying at a deeper emotional level.

However, most of us, as we matured, developed habitual perceptual patterns which directly block our simple enjoyment of seeing. We are so busy using our eyes to perform visual tasks, we forget to pause and take a breather and enjoy ourselves visually.

What about your own case? How many minutes or hours a day do you estimate you spend in simple enjoyment of perception? Naturally, in the modern world most of us lead hectic lives, so we are not free to enjoy our perceptions much of the time. But have we lost most of our ability to shift out of the survival-motivated habits of perception, into the enjoyment-motivated states? Are we in fact manic with our visual habits, not stopping to relax and allow the eyes to look and enjoy what they want to for a few minutes every hour or so?

We are also frightened of what might happen if we allowed ourselves to slip into this somewhat hedonistic state of perception. Especially in the Protestant tradition, it is considered somewhat of a sin against God to spend time doing nothing. Hence we may still feel we should be at work at something all the time, without our hands being idle.

Survival certainly comes first. We must use our eyes as workers to perform the necessary tasks of making a living, taking care of families, etc. But conversely, if we never pause to stop and look at the beauty of life, what is it that we are living for anyway? If simple perception can make us feel better, more in harmony with nature, perhaps we should take more advantage of it.

We tend to forget just how great an alteration we went through when we started school. Before school, our eyes were mostly free to do whatever thay wanted to do. They were not forced to perform reading tasks, writing tasks, for hours a day. They could just look around as they wanted to, absorbing the environment, learning, but also enjoying the process.

Pleasure and enjoyment are emotional states. They are directly related to our conditioning, to our instinctual expressions, and to our breathing patterns. Pleasure takes place in time and space. If we hurry too fast, we lose our sense of enjoyment of life. If the struggle for survival presses in on us with anxiety and worries, we likewise cannot enjoy ourselves. It is impossible to be caught up in fear and to experience pleasure at the same time.

Fear is a contradiction of our awareness. Enjoyment is an expansion. So to the extent that we are anxious, we are not free to enjoy ourselves, visually or in other ways. If we are under stress and hurrying faster than we can go without losing ourselves in calculations and future plans, then we have lost the dimension of pleasure from our perceptual lives.

BREATHING AND VISUAL PLEASURE

We can take a look at our breathing and at our vision patterns, in order to evaluate our perceptual pleasure potential. Pleasure requires a relaxing of the breathing, so that tensions are relieved and good feelings can flow through the body. For the next four breaths, just sit with your eyes closed and watch how you are breathing. Is your breathing tight and high in your chest, focusing on the inhalation? Or is your breathing deep and focused on the exhalation, expansive and relaxed? Just watch for four breaths without altering the breathing at all. See how you are in fact breathing right now.

THE PERCEPTION OF BEAUTY

Primarily, if we want to enjoy the sensory experience of seeing, we need to quiet the judging, labelling, categorizing, conceptualizing parts of our consciousness, and simply allow the visual inputs to come into the brain and be appreciated as a direct stimulation from the outside reality.

Seeing should at times be like tactile feeling. In the same way that a feather drawn lightly across your skin can feel remarkably good in itself, seeing something existing on this planet of ours can be a direct sensory stimulation as well. We can look at the sunset, or the leaves blowing in a gentle breeze, or someone's eyes, and see pure nature, see what is actually there in reality, rather than activating the conceptual processes of the mind.

This is, of course, the basic form of meditation, this simple looking to see what is there, without 'doing' anything with the perception. A simple perception can touch us deeply, beyond thoughts. We can be 'moved' by the beauty of nature, or overwhelmed by the patterns of a Persian rug. A skyscraper can strike us with its grandeur, and a playing kitten can make our hearts sing – all through simple perception matched with breath awareness and an enhanced awareness of our emotions and bodies.

When we explored the four modes of seeing in Chapter 2, we were laying the groundwork for the pleasure of seeing. We can carry on with that discussion now.

In looking to see movement, we quickly determine if we are in danger, or if there is something we should be dealing with in our immediate environment.

By looking to see form, we explore the symbolism and relatedness of what we are looking at, with our past experiences and inner realms of intuition. The eyes naturally enjoy moving around the periphery of an object, taking it in with hundreds of pictures.

Then the experience of colour comes to us, as we move out of our conceptual minds even more, and allow the vibratory quality of an object to stimulate us directly.

And finally we come to the critical point in visual pleasure – perception of three dimensions, of depth, of the reality of expanded life on planet Earth. How do you do with this last way of seeing? Can you look to see everything at once, or are your eyes so used to scanning and taking in detail, that it seems impossible simply to relax and experience everything coming into your visual centre at once, with equal value, with no specific focus on a point?

Look around the room now for four breaths, and see how your eyes naturally want to see what is around you, when you make no effort.

Learning to enjoy the process of seeing is not just a hedonistic pursuit, although there is certainly nothing wrong with experiencing pleasure for its own sake. But this relaxed, pleasurable mode of seeing also serves to revitalize the visual system. It brings life back into the tired optic realms, and links your emotions with your seeing more directly.

Certainly not everything you look at is beautiful. There is a level of perception which is one step more expanded than looking to see beauty. This is the simple looking without any judgement at all, an acceptance of the world as it is, in its totality.

Try looking in this non-judgemental way for four breaths. Just look around the room and allow your eyes to look at everything at once, at anything without preference, and breathe into whatever you encounter, without rejecting anything. Try it now.

Can you experience yourself here right now in space through looking around you and being conscious of yourself at the same time you are conscious of external objects? We tend to lose our awareness of ourselves when we focus on something in our environment. But an integration of our self-awareness with our awareness of the world outside enables us to tap the vitality and life-force we have inside us, if we only will let it come out and enjoy itself!

10 · REVIEW AND PROGRAMME

This final chapter of Part One offers you seven different programmes to choose from, depending on the time you have available, your particular interests and visual needs, and your freedom of movement in the present environment.

First, a review of the exercises, chapter by chapter, is given, so you can quickly see what you have learned so far, and use this list for exploring the exercises by topic. There are thirty-four exercises in Part One, along with suggestions for dealing with specific visual situations.

Seven exercise programmes are then outlined, with accompanying illustrations to remind you instantly of how to do them:

1. The two-minute energizing programme
2. The five-minute vitality programme
3. The ten-minute visual performance programme
4. The ten-minute relaxation programme
5. The fifteen-minute holistic programme
6. The half-hour total visual health programme
7. Your own preference of programme contents

With these guidelines, you should be able to enjoy these exercises easily.

REVIEW OF PART ONE EXERCISE PROGRAMME

Chapter 1

	Page		Page
1. Circle perception	12-13	4. Blinking habits	16-17
2. Healthy reading habits	13-14	5. Tracking/visual shifting	18-22
3. Focal shifting exercise	16	6. The palming meditation	23

Chapter 2

7. Perception of movement	26	10. Perception of volume/space	28-9
8. Form perception	27	11. Perceptual integration exercise	31
9. Aesthetic perception – colour	27		

Chapter 3

12. Image visualization   32-3, 37
13. Movement visualization – bird   34
14. Colour visualization – sky   35
15. Visualization of volume
     space   35-6

16. Remembering childhood
     home/parents   36
17. Visualizing your own face   36

Chapter 4

18. Stretching; yawning   44-5
19. Neck rolls; reverse
     gravity hanging   45
20. Head stimulation; long swings   46
21. Fencer's stretch:
     accommodation   46

22. Jumping; charging;
     running   47-8
23. Pelvic rock   48-9
24. Shoulder stand; palming
     meditation   49

Chapter 5

25. Personal power;
     vocalization   52-3
26. Fear/assertion exercise   54

27. The inner smile   55
28. Facing your danger   55-6

Chapter 6

29. Whole body relaxation   57-8
30. Tension/relaxation exercise   58-9
31. Eye massage and acupressure   59

32. Guided relaxation session   59-60
33. Facial relaxation/palming   60-61
34. Breathing through the eyes   61

VISUAL HEALTH EXERCISE PROGRAMME (PART ONE)

As a beginning, you will want to explore the exercises as they relate to the discussion of your general visual health. This means that you will take a chapter at a time, and do the exercises included in that chapter. Each chapter will give you a particular dimension of visual health:

1. *Muscular co-ordination*
2. *Enhanced perception*
3. *Visualization ability*
4. *Whole-body vitality*

5. *Perception and emotions; assertion*
6. *Relaxation techniques*

You can glance at this list, and your eyes will be attracted to a particular title. Respond to this natural interest, and turn to that chapter for an exercise session.

     Each of these sections of exercises will take you approximately fifteen minutes to complete. This means that you need set aside only fifteen minutes a day for your exercises, and in a week, you will have completed them all.

After two weeks of this complete visual health programme, you can then do the alternative programmes suggested in the following pages. Or if you have a specific vision problem, do the programmes suggested in Part Two.

The Two-Minute Energizing Programme

For an instant regaining of vitality in the body and the eyes, you can stand anywhere and do the following exercises:

		Page
1.	Stretching; yawning	44-5
2.	Neck rolls; reverse gravity hanging	45
3.	Jumping; charging	47-8

Be sure to focus on your breathing and your eyes as you do these movements, so that your conscious awareness helps in the energizing process.

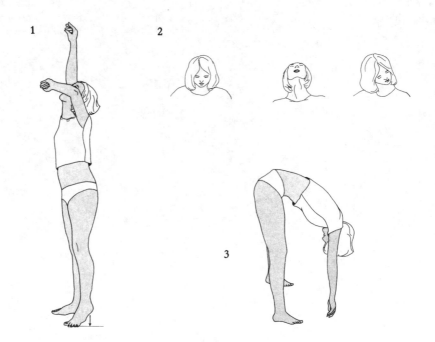

The Five-Minute Vitality Programme

To combine physical vitality with emotional release and increased personal power, both in the body and the eyes, do the following order of exercises:

		Page
1.	Stretching; yawning	44-5
2.	Head stimulation; long swings	46
3.	Fencer's stretch	46
4.	Fear/assertion exercise	54

Allow an increased sense of energy to flow through the eyes as you do these exercises, and expand your breathing to mobilize your visual assertion.

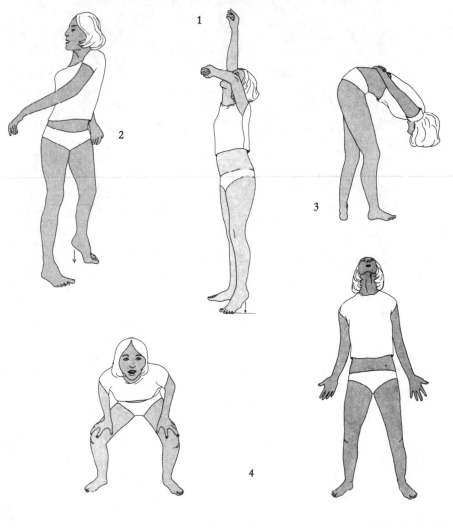

The Ten-Minute Visual Performance Programme

At least once a week, you will want to go through these exercises, to make sure that your visual performance is improving and that your eye habits are also developing positively:

		Page
1.	Eye massage; relaxation	59
2.	Focal shifting (accommodation)	16
3.	Perceptual integration	31
4.	Image visualization	32-3, 37
5.	Palming meditation	23

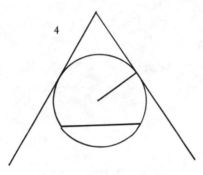

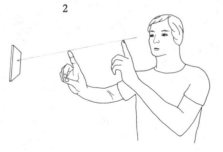

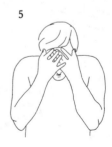

The Ten-Minute Relaxation Programme

Perhaps every day, you should give your body, your mind, and your eyes a break, through focusing completely on muscular relaxation and visual relaxation, along with mental quiet and peace:

		Page
1.	Stretching; yawning	44-5
2.	Neck rolls; reverse gravity hanging	45
3.	Personal power; vocalization	52-3
4.	Pelvic rock	48-9
5.	Whole-body relaxation	57-8
6.	Facial relaxation; palming	60-1

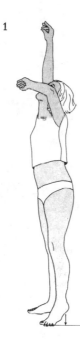

1

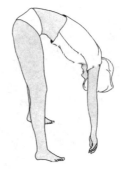

3

2

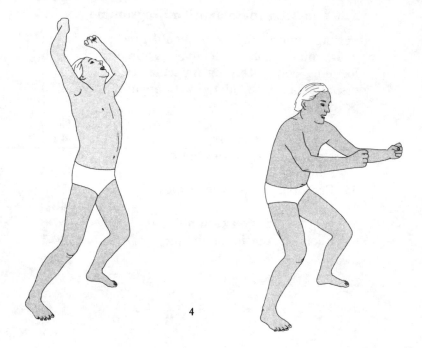

4

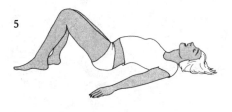

5

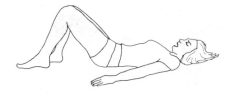

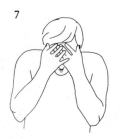

7

The Fifteen-Minute Holistic Programme

This series of exercises combines all the aspects of visual health into one session, bringing your mind's attention to each of the various dimensions of vitality and perceptual performance:

		Page
1.	Stretching; yawning	44-5
2.	Head stimulation; long swings	46
3.	Fear/assertion exercise	54
4.	Tracking/visual shifting	18-22
5.	Perceptual integration	31
6.	Visualizing your own face	36
7.	Pelvic rock	48-9
8.	Whole-body relaxation	57-8
9.	Breathing through the eyes	61

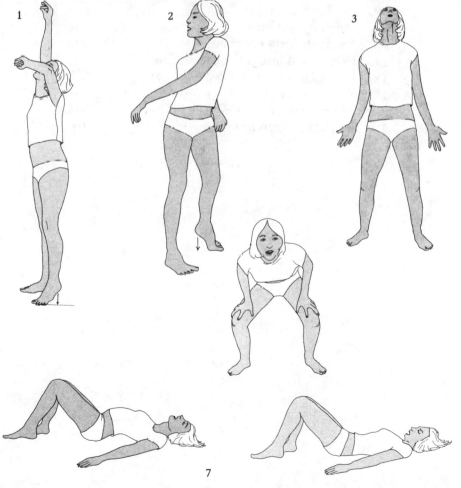

The Half-Hour Total Visual Health Programme

At least once a week, give yourself a full half-hour, and enjoy this series of exercises. As with the other programmes, there is a cassette recording to guide you through this session if you desire that external encouragement:

		Page
1.	Stretching; yawning	44-5
2.	Neck rolls; reverse gravity hanging	45
3.	Jumping; charging; running	47-8
4.	Pelvic rock	48-9
5.	Shoulder stand; palming	49
6.	Head stimulation; long swings	46
7.	Personal power; vocalization	52-3
8.	Fear/assertion exercise	54
9.	Fencer's stretch/accommodation	46
10.	Focal shifting exercise	16
11.	Perceptual integration exercise	31
12.	Visualization practice	32-7
13.	The inner smile	55
14.	Tension/relaxation	58-9
15.	Breathing through the eyes	61

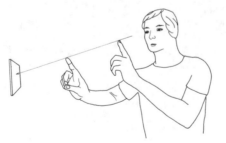

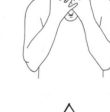

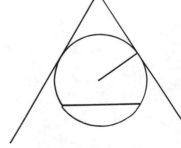

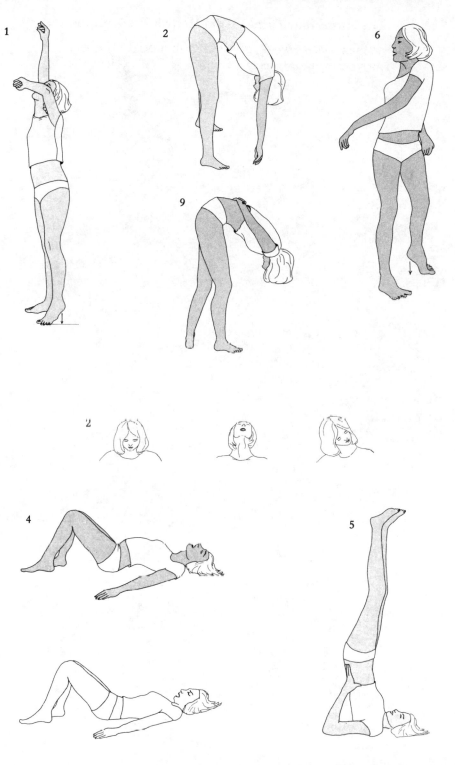

7

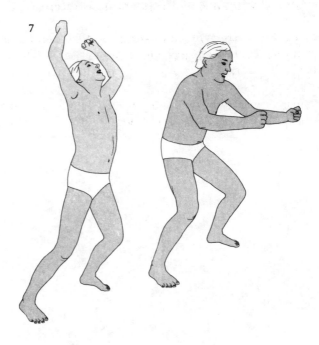

8

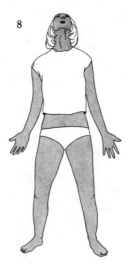

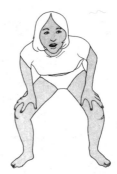

Your Own Preference of Programme Contents

Once you know the various exercises, feel free to develop your own programme. Each of the exercises has a special value, and the ones you are naturally attracted to and enjoy doing will be those which are most important to you at the time.

So once a month or so, make your own list of the exercises you want to focus on for the next thirty days.

PART TWO
Visual Treatment
and Recovery Programmes

INTRODUCTION
When Problems Appear

The seven visual complications which are discussed in this section are the most common eye problems in our culture. Over 60 per cent of us suffer from one or the other of these conditions. Some of the complications, such as crossed eyes and eye allergies, are often present very early in our lives, and myopia usually develops during childhood as well. Others, such as far-sightedness and cataracts, tend to develop after the age of 50.

I hope that you will read the discussions for each of the visual problems, regardless of your particular condition. You will find very interesting similarities between the different vision conditions, and gain a deeper overall picture of how our eyes, our minds, our emotions, our genetic inheritance, and our physical health combine to generate particular complications in the visual system.

There are no miracle cures for vision problems, but there are practical steps you can take, both medical and non-medical, to help yourself. I wish you success with your particular challenge of visual recovery and health!

Vision is a holistic enterprise. Only by considering all dimensions of vision can improvement be brought about. What is crucial is the expansion of the mind–eye interaction. And you will experience directly that the exercises in Part One are potent in this activation of mind–eye communication.

The author would appreciate any feedback you might offer regarding your success with this programme!

11 · NEAR-SIGHTEDNESS (MYOPIA)

Myopia is one of the most common eye problems in our society, striking at least one in five of us before we reach the age of 21. Because the incidence of myopia is increasing with every decade that goes by, a serious focus on the causes of such visual deterioration seems essential.

CAUSES

Traditionally, myopia has been treated as a genetic weakness, an unavoidable development inherent in the growth of a child. It was assumed that the outer layers of the eyeball were hereditarily weak, and that the stretching of the eye into an elongated shape was a natural occurrence for a certain percentage of the population.

It does appear valid to associate myopia with a change in the shape of the eyeball. Direct measurement of the distance from the outer surface of the cornea to the surface of the retina does demonstrate that myopic eyes are longer than normal eyes, causing the visual image to come into focus somewhere in front of the retina rather than directly on it.

However the assumption that this altered shape of the eyeball is a purely hereditary development has not proven valid. There seem to be numerous other contributory factors. A look at these will give us a starting point in discussing methods of correcting myopic conditions, and perhaps of helping to prevent the next generations from having to develop the condition at all.

Studies of various populations throughout the world have shown that myopia occurs with different frequencies in different cultures and environments. For instance, people who live a simple peasant life in rural areas are relatively free of myopic complications, with less then 5 per cent of the population needing glasses. People who live in cities and who are well-educated participants in the complexities of contemporary civilization show a marked increase in myopia. A recent study of a graduating class of college seniors showed that over 50 per cent of them had developed myopic difficulties.

Purely genetic factors could not account for such a difference in the incidence of myopia. Furthermore, the constantly increasing rate of myopia amongst a general population over a period of less than seventy-five years cannot be explained by any genetic-causation theory.

Recently, scientists have explored the environmental factor in myopia. Over the last hundred years there have certainly been definite changes in how we use our eyes. In the past, most people were outside much of the time, looking into the distance regularly, and not performing many close-up visual tasks. This has been completely reversed in recent history. Most of us now spend most of our time indoors, looking up-close most of the time.

It has been suggested that this up-close looking generates abnormal pressures in the eye, thus causing the back of the eyeball to stretch out of shape.

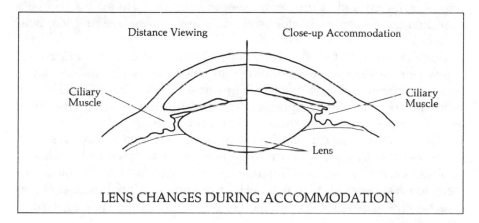

Distance Viewing   Close-up Accommodation

Ciliary Muscle   Ciliary Muscle

Lens

LENS CHANGES DURING ACCOMMODATION

Curious research was done to prove this theory. Several chimpanzees were strapped to chairs and forced to look at a very close visual field for days and even weeks on end, without a break. Thus held prisoner in extremely cruel conditions, the chimpanzees did in fact develop myopic eyesight. However, the emotional strain of the condition was a factor that could also have led to the visual distortion, so the research reached no specific conclusions regarding environment and vision.

Diet has been explored as a cause of myopia. Numerous research projects have tried to locate a correlation between poor diet and visual failure, without success. It was noted that myopic people have a tendency to lowered blood calcium, but dietary alterations of this factor did not influence vision.

The final factor to be considered is that of emotional stress related to physical complications. We know that stress can generate numerous health problems, such as heart attacks, high blood pressure, ulcers, headaches and backaches, allergic reactions, and chronic muscle tension. To what extent would negative emotional states generate a loss of clear vision?

This appears to be the most important question to be answered in the next phase of myopia research. At the present moment, we can look to existing studies which give credence to the psychological factor in myopia.

For instance, myopic people tend to have similar personality traits. As a group, they are more introverted, are inhibited in their expression of anger, move less, interact less with social groups, and show a general emotional inhibition which distinguishes them from the non-myopic population.

Myopic people tend to be inflexible in their attitudes, show a reduction in emotional spontaneity, have a high mental speed, and are more self-centered than non-myopic people. They are socially dominant, intellectually focused, and are over-attracted to near objects.

Such personality tests are only general guidelines, but they do reveal a relationship between particular inhibitions at the emotional level, and a tendency towards myopia. The question remains: did the loss of visual clarity develop the personality traits, or did existing emotional constrictions lead to a change in visual functioning?

Questions such as this one have not been answered as yet. Research is extremely difficult with myopia, because it is often impossible to isolate variables and to focus on just one factor. In fact, the relationship between visual functioning and emotional/mental states has barely been explored at all, and remains a frontier requiring serious inspection.

But certain conclusions can be reached at this point, which help us in devising practical treatment for myopia, and also point towards the possibility of visual recovery. First of all, rather than trying to isolate one cause of myopia, it is obvious that several factors together lead to near-sightedness. The genetic factor is of course an ever-present influence on any bodily function. Environmental stress certainly puts strain on the visual system. And emotional stress is documented as generating alterations in physical functioning throughout the body.

When we take a closer look at the differences between a myopic eye and a normal eye, we see that three variables could lead to blurred distance vision. Elongation of the eyeball, as already shown, is one factor. The second would be the functioning of the lens in focusing the light on the retina. If the ciliary muscles are chronically tense, it is impossible to focus in the distance, because the lens cannot flatten enough to do this focusing.

Perhaps myopic people simply have overly-tense ciliary muscles which make distance viewing impossible. This was considered, but research proved this factor unimportant. Through putting eye-drops in the eyes which relaxed the ciliary muscles for a period of time, inspection could be made to see if the vision now functioned normally with distance vision. In fact, even with the ciliary muscles relaxed and the lens in proper shape for distance vision, myopic conditions remained.

The tension in the ciliary muscles can indeed cause 'pseudo-myopia', and optometrists regularly check for this condition before prescribing corrective lenses. Only in a few cases is blurred distance vision a simple factor of ciliary tension. Usually, the shape of the eye-ball is also causing the loss of distance vision.

There is one other possibility for improper focusing in the eyes. This is the curvature of the cornea, which determines over 70 per cent of the focusing power of the eyes.

Most of us already know how contact lenses alter the curvature of the cornea. With the new soft lenses in particular, very slight alterations in the refractive curve of the cornea generate total correction of myopic vision. This means that any change in the natural curve of the cornea would seriously alter the focusing ability of the eye.

Traditionally, the cornea has been seen as a constant. The collagen fibres in the cornea have been considered inelastic, maintaining a constant curve on the outer surface of the eye. But recent research into their nature indicates that they are in fact elastic in the sense that they alter their length in response to bio-chemical changes within the cornea.

In addition recent studies indicate that the cornea changes its curvature slightly all the time, suggesting that greater alterations, over time and under emotional stress which changes the bio-chemical functioning of the body, could be a factor in both the development of myopia, and also in the reversal of the condition towards visual recovery.

Although professionals hate to admit it, we simply do not understand the causal factors in myopia. The deeper we look, the more complex the picture becomes. Numerous theories exist, but none of them stands as a proven hypothesis. Our concepts of how we function are not sophisticated enough to reflect the reality we are attempting to understand. This is, in fact, the situation in most scientific circles at the present moment. The more we know, the more there is to know.

The current ophthalmological model of myopia, for instance, states that the shape of the eyeball is not elastic. This means that once it stretches out of shape, there is no hope of reversing this process and bringing it back to normal.

However, numerous myopic people, the author included, have sucessfully recovered completely from myopia, demonstrating that somehow, the eye did correct its shape. The mechanics for this correction are not yet known, but the possibility has been demonstrated.

Also, most myopic people periodically experience flashes of clear vision, if they rest their eyes for a period of time. These flashes of momentary clarity indicate that the eye has the ability to correct the myopic distortion, but that as soon as this correction occurs, a habitual reflex returns the eyes to their distorted shape.

One school of thought theorizes that the extraocular muscles which surround the eyes can influence the shape of the eyes. If tensions are generated in these muscles, the shape of the eye would be altered. This has not been proven, but it remains one variable which could in fact influence the myopic condition.

This muscle tension, of course, is linked directly with emotional states. In chronic anxiety or stress, these muscles are affected along with the general musculature of the body.

Many researchers are now taking a step back from the strictly medical approach to the eyes, and are gaining a perspective which could provide the breakthrough in myopia treatment, prevention, and recovery. This new perspective assumes that the changes in the functioning and shape of the eyes take place because, at some emotional level, the brain has determined that it is to the advantage of the organism to make that change.

This means that children unconsciously distort their visual functioning, because this enables them to survive more successfully. Instead of seeing myopia as a disease which strikes an innocent victim, this new approach to myopia assumes that the body is making alterations for a positive reason.

Why would it be to the advantage of a child to eliminate the ability to see the world around him or her?

Childhood is full of trauma, fears, anxiety and stress. No matter how successfully parents nurture their children, there is always conflict, punishment of some sort, inhibitions of instinctual expressions, and imaginary fears.

Fear generates a state of stress and arousal in the body. If the person can release that charge of energy through either attacking or running away from the danger, then tension is discharged, the fear is eliminated, and all is well again.

But what happens when a child is in a situation which generates fear, tension, and anxiety, but which cannot be dealt with through action and resolution? What happens when the fear state maintains constant stress in the body?

Basic physiological research in stress and fear shows that prolonged stress jeopardizes health — and even survival. We naturally try to reduce stress whenever we can, and to cope with it so that constant tension is not maintained in the body.

A child lives in an environment which generates fear. It cannot always run away from the danger, nor can it attack and eliminate it. What is the next possibility for reducing the constant tension?

For a little child, if it cannot see something, then the object does not exist. Myopia is very possibly a regression back to this level of perception. If the child cannot act to eliminate or escape from the threat, them the only remaining step would be to alter the visual functioning so that the danger disappears through a visual elimination.

Thus, developing a distorted eyeball would serve a practical – and for the child perhaps even an essential – purpose. By blurring away the outside world, the danger is seemingly eliminated. Myopia might be a retreat away from a danger through perceptual distortion.

In fact, through years of therapy work with myopic people, the author and his colleagues have found this theory to stand firm. Adults who have been short-sighted since childhood do demonstrate a tendency to avoid looking towards anything which upsets or frightens them. And childhood memories invariably include situations, imaginary fears, or threatening people who generated the escape impulse in the child.

If we approach myopia as an unconscious decision of the brain to distort the visual functioning, then we can integrate the various theories of myopia into one inclusive model.

The brain has a problem to solve. Every time the child looks out at the environment, the possibility exists that a threatening danger might be seen. Even the anticipation of encountering this visual threat generates anxiety, and the stress of this constant arousal in the body is dangerous to the health of the child.

So the brain analyses the problem, sees that nothing can be done to remove the danger, nothing can be done in terms of physically running away from the danger. But a third alternative is in fact possible. By somehow blurring the vision, the danger will disappear. From all perceptual levels, the danger will then be gone and stress will be reduced.

So from this positive approach, how could the brain bring about distortions in the vision to blur the eyesight?

Certainly, ciliary tension would temporarily blur distance viewing. But as soon as relaxation occurred, visual clarity would resume and the danger would be visually present again. So that solution would not work.

A change in the functioning of the eye muscles would help. If tension freezes the eyes, less visual information will be received. In fact, such tension almost always accompanies myopia.

In the longer term, however, changing the shape of the eyeball and increasing the curvature of the cornea are the two alterations which would be most effective in blurring the outside world.

How the brain interacts with the cellular functioning of the body is not yet understood clearly, and involves a vast realm of exploration which will take decades to resolve in even the most simple terms. But the fact remains that the sclera of the eyeballs does stretch, and the eyeball does become elongated. The curvature of the cornea changes as well.

We now have a practical, reasonable working model for the development of myopia. It is the most inclusive model available, and it integrates psychological factors into the medical factors beautifully.

But a further question must now be considered: if the brain ordered such changes to develop, is it possible for the brain to reverse that development?

The newly emerging visual recovery techniques centre on this question. Because certain people have indeed recovered their clear eyesight after years of myopia, the answer to the question appears to be definitely yes. But how the activation of this reversal occurs remains controversial. Most people who recover their clear eyesight do so while going through emotional therapy, or spontaneously, rather than while optometric studies are being conducted on their corneal curvature or eye shape. So data is unavailable except at the questionnaire level.

What is certain is the following: the first step in the recovery of clear vision must be an emotional healing of the contractions and fears which generated the need for distorted vision in the first place. Therefore, visual recovery is part of a general emotional recovery which includes facing your fears and buried childhood reactions to the outside world. Only when you consciously choose to see clearly again, and break through the unconscious habits which maintain emotional contraction and physical distortion, can visual recovery take place.

Before presenting such a programme, we should consider the existing medical techniques for dealing with myopia, so that you can get a good feeling of which approaches ring true for your particular condition.

OPTOMETRIC TREATMENT OF MYOPIA

When a child or young adult is discovered to have failing distance vision, the usual treatment is to go to the optometrist to obtain a pair of corrective glasses. We should not in any way reject or reduce the value of this means of dealing with the symptoms of myopia. It is marvellous that we can see clearly through glasses, when our natural eyesight has become distorted. Optical correction of myopia might not cure the condition, but it does effectively treat the symptom, and enable myopic people to function normally.

Let us briefly explore the process involved in the determination of your prescription for glasses.

Equipment for visual testing has become extremely complex, but basically, in measuring myopic distortion, the purpose of such equipment is straightforward. The tests determine what type of external lens is required in order to bring your visual focus to a point directly on the retina, rather than in front of it as occurs without correction.

Visual tests also determine if your cornea has a consistent curvature, or if there are distortions to this outer lens which require corrections in the external glasses. Improper curvature of the cornea is called astigmatism, and is responsible for the condition of multiple image. For instance, when you look at the moon or at lights at night, improper curvature of the cornea will generate double images, or 'ghost images' as they are often called. This condition can be at least partially corrected through external lenses.

Once your eyes have been measured and a prescription determined for your eyes, you simply choose what frames you want to wear, or if you are going to use contact lenses. Wearing glasses in front of your eyes corrects your clear distance vision, but causes distortions when you turn your head, and a loss of peripheral vision. Contact lenses eliminate this secondary distortion, but often cause irritation of the eyes.

The specifics of contact lens wearing are quite complex these days, and you can obtain a complete explanation from your optometrist upon request.

Complications in Optometric Treatment

If visual acuity is considered a purely physical phenomenon, uninfluenced by emotions, then the visit to the optometrist is quite simple. However, the emotional effects on vision are important and noticeable, and interfere with the measurement of visual acuity.

For instance, fear reduces visual performance, and generates complex reactions throughout the perceptual system. Visual measurements vary depending on the emotional state of the patient. Therefore, if you are anxious when you are being tested, your eyesight will appear to be worse than it normally is, and you will receive glasses which are too strong for you.

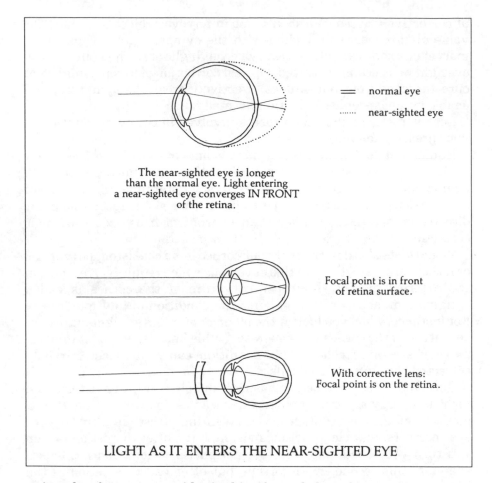

The near-sighted eye is longer
than the normal eye. Light entering
a near-sighted eye converges IN FRONT
of the retina.

= normal eye

...... near-sighted eye

Focal point is in front
of retina surface.

With corrective lens:
Focal point is on the retina.

LIGHT AS IT ENTERS THE NEAR-SIGHTED EYE

Another factor to consider is this: if you do have hopes of improving your eyesight, wearing glasses which eliminate the symptom will make it impossible for your vision to improve naturally. If your brain is receiving inputs which tell it that everything is functioning correctly, there will be no impetus for visual correction to occur.

Only when your blur exists in the distance, does your brain detect a problem in the visual functioning, and only then can possible alterations occur to improve eyesight.

Therefore, it is recommended that you get glasses which are reduced one diopter (a technical measurement of the focal power of your eyes) from the normal prescription for clear vision. You can still drive with this reduction, but distance vision will be slightly blurry, leaving room for improvement.

You will also notice that, if your eyesight improves when you are not wearing your glasses, that as soon as you put your glasses back on, your eyes have to correct negatively in order to adjust to the strength of the glasses. So you will defeat any efforts at improvement if your glasses are full-power.

Wearing contact lenses further confuses your brain's interpretation of your visual condition, because with contact lenses, there is almost no realization that any correction device exists in front of the eyes. You can at least have a one-diopter reduced presciption for your lenses also, and wear your glasses periodically to maintain a conscious awareness of your visual condition.

Of course, if vision improvement is not important to you, glasses and contact lenses are a perfect solution to the symptoms of myopia. Only if you want to improve your vision, are reduced-prescription lenses suggested.

If your optometrist does not want to give you a reduced-prescription, simply phone different optometrists until you find one who agrees with the principle, and who is happy to write you the reduced (one diopter) prescription.

Naturally, as your vision improves, you will need to get even further-reduced prescriptions. This is an unavoidable expense in most cases, unless your vision recovery is very rapid.

SURGICAL ATTEMPTS AT MYOPIA CORRECTION

Experimental surgery has been performed in a number of different countries, most notably in the Soviet Union and the United States, to correct myopic conditions. Although there are no surgical techniques which appear successful at the moment, it is possible that, from a purely physiological level, this approach offers hope in the future.

The techniques vary, but basically the approach is to alter the curvature of the cornea, to flatten it slightly, so that the focal power of the eye is reduced, and the image lands in focus on the retina.

Complications abound, and there are hundreds of people going around with extremely unusual corneas as a result of surgery techniques. One of the techniques is to make incisions in the cornea as shown in the illustration overleaf, leaving the central section of the cornea untouched, but slicing the periphery in such a way as to flatten the central portion.

The results of this surgery technique give us a general insight into the difficulties of even successful operations to correct myopia.

In the Soviet Union, such surgery temporarily corrected the myopic condition, at least partially, for most of the clients. But within months, and sometimes weeks, the correction deteriorated back to the original blurred vision.

Curiously, about 20 per cent of the operations did not exhibit this deterioration. It was found that a particular personality type

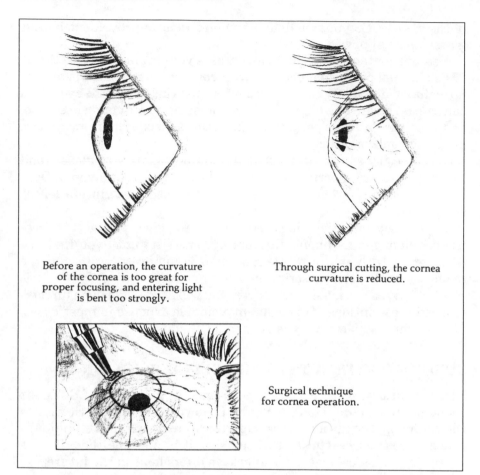

Before an operation, the curvature
of the cornea is too great for
proper focusing, and entering light
is bent too strongly.

Through surgical cutting, the cornea
curvature is reduced.

Surgical technique
for cornea operation.

maintained relatively clear vision, at least for a longer period of time. This personality type was relatively free of the personality traits listed earlier in this chapter, and would therefore be ready emotionally for the visual recovery.

But for the others, at some deep level, the surgical elimination of the visual problem was not accepted, and the correction was reversed back to the myopic state.

This raises an important ethical point which surgeons need to consider. If a person has developed myopia as a defence against emotional trauma, what happens them the myopic defence is eliminated surgically? The person is suddenly without the perceptual defence, and will be subjected to unexplored psychological turmoil which needs to be monitored following the operation.

If we unconsciously chose to blur our vision when we were children, medical attempts to correct that condition will be complicated by the emotional reaction which violates the organism's original decision to generate the blurred eyesight. This is especially crucial for highly myopic people who developed the condition early in childhood.

When we are wearing glasses, we are still hiding behind our crutches. Psychological tests have shown that people respond very differently to emotional images when looking through glass to the way in which they respond when looking directly at the outside world without any glass barrier. Glasses correct visual acuity, but they offer a direct insulation against outside scenes, reducing emotional contact with the visual world. With surgery, this final insulation is removed, and if the person is not emotionally prepared for the sudden return to clear direct perception, trauma will result, and usually a development of further myopia conditions.

Another technique for correcting myopia through surgery is to freeze a removed portion of the cornea, and then to grind down that surface to make it flatter. This is a very precise undertaking, and thus far has not proven successful, even if the returned top of the cornea successfully adheres to the remaining part.

Wedges have also been implanted in the cornea to alter the curvature, with a little success.

From a physiological standpoint, science should one day find a way to succeed with such operations. The question will remain as to whether the emotional constitution of the patient will quickly erode whatever corrections were made.

Hopefully, psychological and medical approaches can be brought together, so that possibilities in both fields can combine to offer a total approach to myopia correction.

ORTHOKERATOLOGY

This long word refers to another experimental technique for flattening the curvature of the cornea in order to reduce myopia. The approach of orthokeratology is to use special contact lenses to bring about this flattening of the corneal surface.

Through wearing contact lenses which are less curved than is the cornea, a flattening process is instigated. Over a period of years, and sometimes months, a full correction of myopia can be generated, usually after progressing through several very expensive pairs of corrective lenses.

Unfortunately, as soon as the special contact lenses are put aside, the corneas begin to return to their original myopic curvature, except in a few cases. This might be a simple physiological return, or the emotional factor which we mentioned already could instigate a return to the original state of blurred vision.

Future research combining orthokeratology and emotional therapy could result in a successful treatment of myopia. Once the deeper dimensions of blurred vision are dealt with, the mechanical reduction in corneal curvature through corrective contact lenses would very possibly accelerate the recovery process.

However, there are additional factors which raise professional reservations regarding orthokeratology; these are briefly explained below.

First of all, wearing the special lenses generates changes in the actual physiology of the cornea. These include changes in contour, homogeneity, lustre, refraction, and sensation. Also, changes have been noticed in the epithelium, lemelle, and thickness of the cornea. The possibility of pathological changes is also present in terms of infection, opacity, and vascularization.

Such potential complications have not been explored fully because long-term studies of orthokeratology do not yet exist.

In summary, orthokeratology is very expensive, takes several years to complete, and usually reverses back to its original blur state if retainer lenses are not worn regularly. Combining this corrective technique with psychological preparation for visual recovery could be a key factor in the future success of the technique.

VISION IMPROVEMENT TECHNIQUES

Vision improvement exercises, as opposed to the more advanced and controversial visual recovery programmes offered later in this chapter, are traditional visual therapy exercises drawn from several optometric and psychological approaches to enhanced visual functioning.

These vision improvement exercises are designed to help you improve your eyesight perhaps 10–25 per cent, with occasional improvements beyond this level. These exercises, most of which have already been introduced in the first part of the book, are the essential first steps upon which the visual recovery programme is based, so you will want to explore fully this series of exercises before moving to the final recovery phase.

It should be stated clearly that these improvement and recovery programmes are experimental, and offer no promise of recovery beyond the fact that they have helped a considerable number of people, and thus have demonstrated their potential. Although sustained by a concrete medical model, the programmes are still beyond the scope of current visual research.

However, there is definitely no danger of complications through exploring these programmes for visual recovery. For those of you who respond to the exercises and healing sessions, the potential for full recovery exists. For those of you with only partial success, the programmes will certainly expand your visual performance and enjoyment, and your general integration of visual functioning into your overall personality.

BASIC SUPPORTING EXERCISES

To complement the specific vision improvement exercises presented in this section, it is highly recommended that you do the following exercise schedule once a day, before beginning the actual vision improvement exercises:

		Page
1.	Stretching; yawning	44-5
2.	Neck rolls; reverse-gravity hanging	45
3.	Head stimulation; long swings	46
4.	Jumping; running.	47-8

And afterwards:
5.	Palming meditation	23
6.	Perceptual integration exercise	31
7.	Whole-body relaxation.	57-8

While doing these exercises, be sure to remain aware of your eyes, and also of your breathing.

As we mentioned before, the myopic personality tends towards reduced movement in daily life, which includes both whole-body movement and also eye-movement. These exercises when done regularly directly act to reverse your habits of inhibited breathing and movement, while also expanding the brain-eye interaction which is vital to visual recovery.

After doing this short exercise programme, you can move onto whichever phase of the vision improvement programme you are presently focusing upon.

Phase One

As we have already seen, myopia is basically a reduced ability to focus in the distance. With your glasses off, you can see objects close to your eyes. But as the distance increases from your eyes, everything becomes more and more blurred, out of focus.

By exploring the experience of consciously shifting your focus from an up-close object to a more distant, blurred object, you can directly bring your brain into contact with the essence of your problem, and thus begin the process of visual correction.

FOCAL SHIFTING (Accommodation)

We have already introduced this exercise on page 16. We will now expand on the technique especially for myopic improvement.

Remove your glasses or contact lenses for all the following exercises, and begin noticing that you live within a bubble of clarity, near to your eyes, where everything is actually in focus. If you look around you, you find that you actually have a bubble of clear vision surrounding you. This bubble of clarity is the starting point in vision improvement.

Rather than trying to see in the distance straight away, the best approach to vision improvement is simply to expand your bubble of clarity one small step at a time. If you continually try to push far out into the distance, you will discourage yourself and also generate emotional fears associated with sudden recovery of total visual clarity.

So the first step is to hold one finger up in front of you, near your eyes so that you can see it with perfect clarity. Be thankful that you can at least see this clearly. Accepting your present visual ability is the essential beginning to visual recovery, because you must grow from your actual present condition in order to make any realistic progress.

As you look at your visually sharp finger, bring your attention to your breathing, and notice if it is tense and shallow, reflecting anxiety and stress, or if it is relaxed and smooth, reflecting readiness for growth and healing.

I have never known anyone to improve his or her eyesight without there being parallel improvements in inhibited breathing patterns. This reflects the emotional dimension of visual performance. So throughout these exercises, keep in mind that each one has been designed to help you both with your vision, and also with your breathing habits. (If you want a more detailed programme for breath recovery, consult my *Responsive Breathing*, which is a companion volume to this one.)

Now that you are aware of both your finger and your breathing, raise the forefinger of your other hand directly beyond the first hand. With a smooth exhalation, shift your focus to this second finger, which for most of you will be near the outer limits of your bubble of clarity. Then inhale as you shift your focus back to the close finger again. Do this several times, shifting into the distance as you exhale, and close focusing as you inhale.

Now, after looking to your distant finger, look beyond this point to an object which is just slightly outside your bubble of clarity. Be sure to exhale deeply and completely as you make this shift into your blur zone. A complete exhalation is essential to expanding your vision into the distance, because it mobilizes your strength, assertiveness, and confidence.

After breathing for one complete cycle with your focus in the distance (only a foot or so into your blur zone at first) inhale your focus back to your distant finger, and then on the next inhalation, return your focus to your up-close finger.

You will find that this slow shifting from distance to near and back again, matched with smooth breathing, is more than just an automatic exercise. It is also a form of meditation. Meditation is not meant in any religious connotation here, but rather as a focusing of your mind's attention to the specific regions of your brain where visual functioning is monitored and controlled.

You should approach this exercise in a state of relaxed enjoyment. Rather than 'trying' to improve your eyesight, simply bring your mind's focus to your present condition, and through regularly shifting from clear to blurry vision, you will activate the inherent correction potential of the brain. Many people approach eye exercises in the wrong state of mind, and thus eliminate their potential for visual recovery. Be sure that you leave yourself open to new experiences and insights, rather than forcing a particular state of mind while doing the exercise. Allow the deeper functioning of your brain to be stimulated through your meditation on this accommodation exercise.

VISUAL RELAXATION

Following a strenuous visual exercise such as the focal shifting, it is important to relax the eyes completely. The palming posture presented on page 23 is the basic exercise for visual relaxation.

Be sure that when you pause with your hands over your eyes as shown in the illustration, you remain aware of your eyes *and* your breathing, at the same time. The simple expansion of your mental functioning, is to link breathing (emotions) with your visual functioning, is a crucial first step in this programme.

There should be an increased sense of enjoyment and contentment when you assume the palming posture. Your eyes are now covered, and they are assured by the presence of your hands that they have no work to do. They can relax with no external dangers threatening to impinge on them.

VISUALISATION OF FOCAL SHIFTING

While still palming, and after six breaths of simple breath/eye awareness, you can exercise your visualization ability through imagining the focal shifting exercise you did earlier, and visualise what you actually saw when you had your eyes open and were looking from near to far. Be sure to breathe with the same pattern as you used with your eyes open in the focal shifting exercise.

These three exercises make up the *phase one* part of the vision improvement programme. You should focus on this first aspect of the programme for perhaps ten sessions before moving on. You can do the exercise almost anywhere, and it only takes a few minutes. So as often as once an hour, you can do this three-part *phase one* session, and in a few days you will begin to master the session, discovering numerous insights about your vision, your breathing, and the relationship between your eyes and your brain.

- focal shifting
- visual relaxation
- visualization

Phase Two

FENCER'S STRETCH/ACCOMMODATION

We now move into the combination of focal shifting, breath awareness, and body movement. Bringing these three factors together has an almost magical effect on the vision, stimulating the process of vision improvement and recovery.

The first exercise has been described on page 46 and is called the fencer's stretch/accommodation movement. Be sure that you notice the breathing pattern for this exercise, because it is a reversal of the *phase one* breathing/accommodation pattern. We are in fact exploring another dimension pf emotion/perception in this fencer's stretch, where you exhale with a downward movement, and inhale with the upward movement of your body.

On the exhale, as you bend over, stress is felt throughout the body, associated with the ciliary muscle tension felt in the eyes. Then, as you stand up with an inhale, your body relaxes, and the relaxation of the ciliary muscles is also encouraged.

Continue watching your big toe or the tip of your shoe through three breathing/movement cycles over one foot.

Then pause with your eyes closed, palm, watch your breathing, and notice how your eyes feel.

Then visualize the exercise you just did, remembering visually what you saw as you performed the movement and held your attention to your foot.

Now turn and look down at your other foot, and continue with the second half of the exercise, just as you did for the first half.

WALL FOCUS

You will find this next exercise one of the more enjoyable ones in the programme. Stand as shown in the illustration, facing an open wall. Continue watching the wall in front of you, as you first fall forwards and lean against the wall with your hands, and rock backwards away from the wall.

Exhale through the mouth as you move towards the wall, and then inhale with relaxation as you move away, giving a little push with your hands to begin the movement away from the wall. Do this slowly, rhythmically, and powerfully.

As you exhale and fall towards the wall, contract your abdomen muscles with power, exhaling completely. This action will force the diaphragm muscles to relax, and because a tense diaphragm muscle is associated with myopia, generating this relaxation through pushing and exhaling through the mouth is vital.

Do this exercise perhaps ten times, and then stand upright, close your eyes, and palm, focusing on your breathing and your eyes.

And then, after perhaps five breaths, begin to visualize what you just experienced as you watched the wall from the shifting focal distance. Match your breathing with the imagined movements and visual shifting.

If at first you can't visualize the exercise, please don't try to force it. Accept that you need to return your focus to this visualization exercise regularly, and simply remain passive as you see, day by day, how your effortless visual memory begins to expand its functioning. This visualization ability needs to be nurtured in most of us, since it was blocked by various childhood inhibitions.

HAND ACCOMMODATION

This final exercise in *phase two* is simple and yet powerful, employing a gesture of the hand to match the shifting of focus from near to far and back again.

Begin by holding one of your hands up in front of you, your palm facing your eyes, and look at your palm.

Now, on the exhale, move your hand down and away from you gracefully, as if welcoming your eyes to venture beyond the hand to look at what lies beyond. You might want to have a favourite picture to look at, or one of the visual meditations shown in this book.

Then, on the next inhalation, shift your focus slowly back to your palm, and bring the palm closer to your face so you can see it very clearly.

Notice especially the beautiful sense of letting go which you can experience as your hand moves down and away and encourages you to look into the distance.

At first, look only a foot or two into your blur zone when you shift into the distance. Look at something that you really want to see. Exhale completely before returning your eyes to look at your palm.

Then close your eyes, palm, breathe, and notice how your eyes feel.

Finally, visualize what your eyes saw while doing this exercise.

- fencer's stretch/accommodation
- wall focus
- hand accommodation

As with *phase one*, do these *phase two* exercises ten times over a period of two or three days, and fully tap their potential.

Phase Three

In this final phase of vision improvement exercises, we are going to explore the specific techniques of a famous ophthalmologist named William Bates, who pioneered numerous aspects of the vision improvement schools. Certain aspects of his theories of myopia have been brought into question by recent research, but much of his work still holds valid in the realm of vision improvement, if not of visual recovery.

Perhaps Dr Bates' most controversial suggestion was that myopic conditions are at least partially caused by chronic tension of the extraocular eye muscles, in particular the oblique muscles surrounding the eyes. He believed that the muscles could actually alter the shape of the eyeball through various tensions and relaxation patterns.

Although it seems to be an oversimplification to blame myopia totally on this extraocular muscle tension, it does appear that vision improvement can be related to the proper functioning of the extraocular muscles. Certainly, chronic tension of these muscles will lead to various difficulties in seeing.

So the following exercises are designed to reduce the extraocular muscle tension in your eyes. The exercises are variations on the basic Bates themes.

LONG SWINGS

This exercise has been described on page 46, so perhaps you have already tried it. There is a magic to this particular movement, with regards to the eyes and surrounding muscles. At first, your eyes will try to hold onto the various objects they see as you swing from one distraction to the other. But at some point, perhaps on your first session, perhaps on the tenth or fifteenth, depending on your personal visual state, you will experience a sudden relaxation in the eyes, as they stop trying to grasp hold of what is 'going by', and simply take in whatever visual information naturally occurs.

Part of the magic of this exercise is certainly in the whole-bodily movements. The turning of the head and neck opens up chronic tensions in that region, tensions related to myopic bodily structures. And the turning also loosens up the pelvic region and lower back, further releasing tensions throughout the body.

So it would be a natural progression for the eye muscles to relax also, and this is what appears to happen with long swings. By remaining aware of your breathing also, you activate a deeper consciousness, one which is relaxed and yet alert, balanced and yet not focused on a point.

So do ten to twenty-five long swings, with your breathing relaxed and deep, your enjoyment of the movement being vital to your overall success in this exercise.

EYE RELAXATION ('breathing through the eyes')

Direct focusing on extraocular relaxation can also improve visual functioning. Chapter 6 provides the basic exercises for this relaxation. The final exercise in that chapter, called 'breathing through the eyes', is an expansion on the Bates techniques, and affords a dramatic reduction in visual tensions. So along with regularly exploring the first exercises in Chapter 6, you might want to focus your attention, every day, to at least one twelve-breath session of 'breathing through the eyes'.

Allow your facial muscles to relax as you do this exercise. Drop any smile you might have that is maintaining tension in the superficial muscles of the face, and allow the 'inner smile' (page 55) to radiate tranquillity throughout your facial muscles.

As you exhale, say to yourself 'relax' very slowly and encouragingly, with your focus on the tensions you feel in your eyes. This verbal linkage with breathing and relaxation will work strongly to your advantage.

Then, after perhaps twelve to twenty-four breaths of 'breathing through the eyes', with them closed, open your eyes and continue with the exercise, inhaling the world around you, and then exhaling your sense of power and presence out into the world. Notice if you feel confident and eager to look at the world around you, or if opening your eyes generates anxiety and tensions.

Peaceful Visualization

The fear of seing something negative or threatening is certainly related to visual tensions and malfunctioning. The impulse to avoid the emotional shock of seeing negative scenes will certainly generate its related physical contractions as well as emotional avoidance patterns. So the habit of expecting the outside world to evoke a contraction pattern needs to be dealt with if you are myopic.

Dr Bates initiated a technique which generated considerable results amongst his clients, and which remains as a valuable vision improvement technique. This was the technique of guided visualization. As with several other of these exercises, working with a cassette recording of the session facilitates the process, but you can also recall the steps in the exercise from memory, and work without external guidance.

Find a quiet place to either lie down or sit comfortably, and close your eyes.

Allow your breathing to become calm, regular, and deep, with a feeling of effortless movement of the air in and out of your lungs.

Let your body relax step by step, as you notice tensions and let them relax, from your feet, to your legs, your pelvis, your back, your chest, your arms, your neck, and your head.

Now that you are feeling very comfortable, relaxed, and calm, imagine that you are sitting on a peaceful warm beach. The sunlight is soft and soothing on your skin, and your breathing is free, deep, and effortless.

You have your eyes closed and can feel the warm radiating sunlight on your closed lids, sending pulsating flows of energy directly into the deeper regions of your brain. This sensation brings an expansive, nurturing feeling throughout your body, as if the sun is providing you with vital healing energy.

Your eye muscles relax step by step as the sunlight penetrates through the tensions and melts the stress from your muscles.

Without opening your eyes, you imagine the surrounding beach and ocean view which you have seen before closing your eyes.

You remember seeing the blue of the sky, the white clouds overhead, the glistening sand, the inviting water with waves lapping gently on the soft sand. Your visual memory is perfectly clear and focused in the distance, and you enjoy the visualization of the safe, secure, welcoming landscape.

Then you have the desire to sit up and look again at the beauty and peace which surrounds you, so you sit up in your imagination, and allow you eyes to open when they want to, without forcing the lids to open until they choose to.

Without your glasses, you find that you can see quite perfectly, with a relaxed sensation in your eyes, and a calm, joyful feeling in your chest and your breathing.

With every inhalation, you take in the beauty which surrounds you as you turn your head and look around. And with every exhalation, you feel your vitality and presence flowing out your eyes, letting the world around you know you are there.

In your imagination, you stand up now, feeling full of a new energy which is eager to run along the beach. Your feet enjoy the cool of the wet sand along the shore. Your breathing is powerful and yet relaxed.

And as you look around you as you run gently along the shore, you can still see far into the distance with perfect clarity. You can feel that this new clarity is related to the feeling of peace, confidence, and power that you have with every breath.

You turn around and walk back to your towel, noticing where it is far in the distance. You can see the book you were reading, your watch on the towel, and other items very clearly from a considerable distance.

And then you see someone walking towards you. At first you might feel apprehension, and you find that your vision instantly becomes blurry.

But you breathe into your habit of contracting, and allow your eyesight to focus on the distance and see the person clearly. It is a person whom you find attractive and friendly, someone who is pleased to share your quiet peace with you.

And you now continue with whatever you might imagine happening, until you feel ready to leave the fantasy and return to alert waking consciousness.

After doing this visualization exercise, you want to open your eyes without expecting any great flashes of visual clarity, but knowing that at some point this might occur. Just accept your present visual ability, and feel the sense of renewed vitality and confidence which came from the visualization. See if you can do this fifteen-minute session three times a week for a month, to explore fully your ability to improve your eyesight through this technique.

- long swings
- breathing through the eyes
- visualization of clarity (beach)

This brings us to the end of the vision improvement section of myopia recovery. You now have three phases to move through, with a total of nine exercises crucial to vision improvement.

Once again, these exercises work for some people but not all, and they have varying degrees of success. Both the emotional and the physiological factors of your personal constitution will determine the effectiveness of these sessions.

Many people go through these exercises once and notice very little progress, but then, upon returning to them a second or third time, make the vital connection which provokes growth. So be patient with yourself, and give yourself time.

VISUAL RECOVERY TECHNIQUES (Myopia)

We now find ourselves face to face with a vital question for human beings in general, as well as people with myopic eyes: can the focused attention of the brain generate corrections in the physiological structure of particular regions of the body?

It has been demonstrated that both hypnotic and yogic techniques can in fact alter the functioning of the body. Trained subjects can reduce the temperature of localized parts of their body (the big toe, the knee, the abdominal region, etc.) and also increase the temperature in the rest of the body. Adept yogis in laboratory situations have slowed down their hearts to rates which seem impossible for survival, have stopped the bleeding of experimental wounds, and exhibited supernormal strength and muscle rigidity.

When we turn to actual diseased states of the body, research becomes much more difficult . Certainly we all know of people with medically 'incurable' diseases who have made seemingly miraculous recoveries. Doctors have long known that a small percentage of their patients exhibit recovery patterns which cannot be explained by medical terms or models.

Certainly, visual recovery is no exception. Although there is no known medical cure for myopia, occasionally people do spontaneously regain perfectly clear eyesight after decades of myopic vision. The author underwent such a recovery, and the present programme is a reflection of the techniques which seemed to make that recovery possible.

As in the vision improvement programme, there are three phases in the visual recovery programme, and you are encouraged to take time with each before moving on to the next. The first phase deals with your understanding of the principles of the recovery model. The second is focused on the psychological/emotional growth that seems required for visual recovery. And the third directly guides you through the cornea restructuring sessions which are at the heart of this approach to visual recovery.

Phase Four: Cornea Restructuring

When we look to see the most direct means of correcting myopia, at the physiological level, it is obvious that reducing the curvature of the cornea is the most practical approach. We have already seen the medical and optometric approaches to reducing this curvature. We are now going to consider how this reduction could take place through internal direction.

The cornea consists primarily of fibres called collagen fibres, which run in layers perpendicular to each other, and thus generate the depth of the cornea. Tiny channels are found throughout the collagen layers, tunnels which bring nutrients to the interior of the cornea.

Thus we can see that if the collagen fibres were elastic, they could alter the curvature of the cornea through contraction or relaxation. And also, if the liquids penetrating the interior of the cornea were to increase or decrease in volume, the curvature would also be affected.

Recent studies indicate that in fact, the collagen fibres of the cornea will respond to different ionic conditions with contraction or expansion, encouraging the hypothesis that at this sub-cellular level, the body can act to generate myopic conditions, and also reverse those conditions to normal vision.

The same is true of the liquid content within the cornea. The membrane which admits or rejects entry into the interior of the cornea functions in accordance with biochemical laws which we are only beginning to understand. But this membrane is definitely a variable which can alter the interior volume and functioning of the cornea itself.

So we ask the question: can the brain send orders to the membrane of the cornea, suggesting an alteration in ionic transfer patterns?

When the condition of myopic vision begins to develop, it is very possible that such orders from the brain generate the distortion which occurs. The emotion of fear is a powerful charge in the body, and it is very possible that this charge could be directed to bring about such changes in the body.

So to reverse the condition of myopia, an equal charge of emotional energy will be needed to empower the brain to send the orders to return the curvature of the cornea to normal, and even possibly to return the shape of the eye to normal also. We will therefore need to work at the emotional level as well as the cognitive/vegetative level, to bring about restructuring of the visual system. This will be the focus of *phase five*.

Visualizing the Cornea

The first step here is to develop a clear picture of what actually needs to happen for visual restructuring to take place. Without such a clear image in the brain, the following sessions will not be potent.

So with the aid of memory, or a tape which you have made of the text below, close your eyes and focus on the following visualization:

> First of all be aware of your breathing, moment to moment, and maintain this awareness as you expand your focus to include your eyes. Allow the air to flow in and out of your lungs with absolutely no conscious effort. Simply watch yourself breathing, and notice the source of your next inhalation.
>
> Feel the air going in and out through your nose, so that you are conscious of the actual sensation of the air as it enters your nose, and leaves it again.
>
> Let this awareness expand now, to include the entire volume inside your skull. You can be directly aware of your brain itself, through simply focusing on the space inside your skull.
>
> Be aware of your body as a whole now, without effort. With every inhale, breathe in life and energy, and with every exhale, breathe out tension and stress. Allow a vibrant quality to expand throughout your body.
>
> And now bring your focus to your eyes.
>
> Be conscious of the actual physical presence of your eyes as they rest behind your eyelids. As you breathe, imagine that you are breathing in and out through your eyes as well as through your nose, so that you become even more conscious of the presence of your eyes in your head.
>
> If you had normal eyes with no myopic distortion, your eyes would be generally round in shape. If you are myopic, your eyes are probably elongated backwards a short distance into the soft fat tissue behind your eyes.
>
> Imagine this shape of your eyes, and actually 'feel' the shape of your eyes in your head right now. Do this without mental effort. Just see what you directly experience when you focus your attention on the physical presence of your eyes in your head.
>
> And be aware of the curvature of your cornea now. The surface of your eyes is a beautiful curve, like a glass dome through which you

see the world outside. See if you can feel this curved surface under your eyelids.

If you want to, you can gently feel your cornea under your closed eyelids, with the tips of a finger, running your fingertip gently over the curve to directly experience it.

Continue being aware of your breathing through all this, noticing if it is smooth, deep and relaxed, or if there is tension in the breathing related to this direct focusing on your eyes. Be gentle with yourself, accepting how you are right now, so that natural growth and recovery can begin.

And now imagine what is happening inside your cornea. Millions of cells and collagen fibres are participating to maintain the shape and functioning of your cornea. Constant exchange with the liquid behind the cornea is bringing nutrients into the cornea, and removing waste products.

Imagine the active, vibrant life which exists inside your cornea.

Continue with your breathing while you feel the dynamic activity of the millions of cellular and sub-cellular beings which constantly perform their duties in order to maintain the structure and health of the cornea.

And feel the organic response of your cornea to the activities of the rest of your body. Especially feel the flow of emotional excitation which moves through the interior of the cornea when you experience changes emotionally.

Just breathe into this feeling of contact with your cornea, with the intricate and constantly-changing variables inside the curved outer surface of your eyes.

Feel the potential for slight alterations within your cornea, alterations which will reduce the curvature of the cornea and improve your eyesight.

And as you continue to watch your breathing also, experience your present readiness for this alteration in the curvature of your cornea. Simply be aware of your present state of emotional motivation in ordering your cornea to begin the restructuring process.

And then relax, enjoy your breathing, and open your eyes when they freely want to open again.

Phase Five: Psychological/Emotional Growth

If this new model for visual recovery is correct, then your attitude to seeing the outside world will be a crucial factor in your ability to heal yourself.

Do you really want to see clearly, to face all the real and imagined fears which you blurred out of existence as a child or young adult? Are you ready to regain your clear eyesight, and in so doing deal with the underlying psychological traumas which generated your myopic condition?

Everyone is in a unique state of psychological health and growth, so only you will know your readiness to recover your eyesight. Only be sure not to push yourself. Visual recovery, when it does happen, is a final phase in emotional healing and personality growth. The wisdom of your deeper self will surely block visual recovery until you are emotionally ready for this step.

It is a radical development to recover clear eyesight, after years of blurred vision. The new clarity reverberates throughout your psychological system.

So just imagine for a moment, what it would be like if you employed the techniques of this programme and suddenly found that you had healed yourself. What would your friends think? How would you feel if you were the first person you knew who was in fact able to bring about such a recovery?

Are you ready for all the repercussions of visual recovery?

The following *phase-five* session is designed to help you explore your psychological habits and inhibitions, so that you can let go of the old fears and repulsions which generated your childhood impulse to blur away the outside world. As we have seen, there is strong reason to suspect that myopia is actually a habit itself, a pattern which the brain maintains as an ongoing defence against outside threats. To change this habitual blur pattern is, of course the purpose of this section.

Find a comfortable place to sit or lie down, and relax for the next fifteen minutes as we explore your eyesight and your emotions.

Turn your attention to your breathing, so we can use changes in your breathing as a direct barometer of your internal responses to various suggestions.

Notice the air going in and out of your nose, feel the sensation of the air as it rushes inside you, and then is blown out again.

Breathe effortlessly, with an honest observance of how you are feeling right now, as we approach your feelings about your eyesight.

Without forethought, see what word comes to mind as you consider the question, 'Do I want to regain clear eyesight?'

Notice your breathing and accept either a positive or a negative answer to the question. You will be doing this same exercise a number of times, and you can see how your feelings change as you grow.

Now let your mind wander into your past memories, as you look back to see what childhood experiences might have caused you to want to blur away the outside world. Breathe consciously, and just see what the first memory is that pops into your head right now, and let that memory expand in any directions that naturally happen.

Stay aware of your breathing, and breathe into any memories you are now experiencing.

What faces did you want to blur away?

What imaginary monsters were you afraid you might suddenly see out there somewhere?

Stay with your breathing as the memories come effortlessly to you.

And now allow yourself to feel the fear and repulsion which you felt as a child or young adult. Be brave and finally face the dangers which you ran away from through blurring them into non-existence.

Turn and face your danger. Exhale as you do so and feel your present strength.

Do those people, those dangers, those fears and monsters still threaten you?

Breathe and feel your strength. Exhale completely and push all your fears out of you.

Now inhale a new feeling towards the outside world. Inhale and feel a new confidence inside you, a new strength with which to face whatever is out there without fear.

Be aware of your eyes, and with every exhalation, breathe out through them in your imagination, sending your personal power out into the world. And with every inhalation, bring more power and confidence into your body.

Consciously choose to let go of past habits which keep fear inside you. Let those old fears die. Let go of them.

Breathe.

Be open to whatever memories, insights, or feelings which begin to rise to the surface now. Breathe into whatever comes, let the feelings come up and out, so that the old wounds heal.

If you feel tears coming, allow them release. If you feel anger, pound on the floor with your hands if you want, and vocalize your feelings. Let the pressure be released finally.

Breathe.

Face what scares you.

Look directly at the danger and see if it still exists. Exhale and feel your strength as you look. Breathe out through the mouth.

Let your deeper wisdom guide you to the memory which needs

healing. Keep your breathing expansive and in touch with your feelings.

Accept whatever comes. Look at yourself, be free of this inner blur zone. Focus on the point of your fear.

And now, when you are ready and finished with this session, you can slowly stretch, allow your eyes to open when they want to, and spend a few moments reflecting on what you just learned about yourself and your eyesight.

Phase Six: Visual Restructuring

If you are to regain clear eyesight, the physical structure of your eyes must be altered slightly. The change required is actually quite slight. But a physical event needs to happen for visual recovery to take place.

There is no way of knowing, at present, when you are ready for this change to take place, except to put yourself in a situation which encourages this shift, and to see if it happens. As mentioned before, scientists do not know how it is that the brain interacts with the eyes to bring about a physical alteration. But because numerous people have experienced this restructuring, there is obviously some inner mechanism which makes it happen.

So phase six offers you guidance in encouraging this visual restructuring. You can do this session as often as twice a day, or as seldom as once a week, depending on your motivation and your schedule. But be sure to do phases four and five as often as you do this session, because all three are vital.

Lie down where you will be comfortable and not disturbed for the next twenty minutes. Be sure you are warm and that your clothes are loose.

Feel the floor or bed under your back, and let your breathing begin to relax as you sink comfortably into the pull of gravity.

Surrender to this complete relaxation as you breathe deeply. Stretch and yawn a couple of times if you want right now, further discharging tensions.

Be aware of the air as it goes in and out your nose. Breathe effortlessly, and observe how your breathing feels with each inhale and exhale.

Expand your awareness to include both your breathing through the nose, and your entire head at once.

With each inhalation, bring energy and light into your body. And with each exhalation, blow out remaining tensions as you express your personal power to the outside world.

Now expand your awareness to include your whole body at once, without effort. Just turn your attention to the whole experience of lying there and breathing. With every breath, allow this effortless awareness to expand.

After your next exhalation, make no effort to inhale, and allow your breathing to remain empty for a moment. Let yourself become hungry for air but make no effort to inhale. Then notice the centre deep down in your abdomen which automatically causes you to breathe, without conscious effort, on your next inhalation.

Continue to breathe in this effortless way.

And now with your awareness including your breathing and your whole body, bring your focus gently and effortlessly to the presence of your eyes in their sockets.

Let your experiences with *phase four* enhance your present awareness of your eyes, their shape, vitality, functioning. Be aware of your eyes as living organs, in direct neurological contact with your brain right now.

Breathe effortlessly as this awareness grows, so that you can almost feel the constant neurological communications flowing from your brain to your eyes, and the feedback which the eyes send to the brain.

Feel deeply into those parts of your brain where control of the eyes takes place. Make no effort, simply allow your awareness to expand into these usually unconscious realms of the brain.

Breathe into the expanding feeling of connection between your mind and your eyes.

And now allow your desire to improve your vision to grow as a feeling in your body. Don't force this, simply breathe and see what energy exists in you, right now, to bring about changes in the physical shape and functioning of your eyes.

Feel this desire to see clearly as an actual neurological charge running from the base of your spine, up into your brain, and then allow that charge to flow out to your eyes themselves, carrying direct messages from the brain to bring about visual recovery.

With every breath, let this flow of healing energy and concrete information flow up through you, and out from your brain to your eyes.

To whatever extent you are ready to right now, allow the shape of your eyes to move in the direction of clear vision.

Allow the curvature of your cornea to move in the direction of clear vision.

Let the healing take place right now.

Breathe into the process you are choosing to activate.

Feel the intimate interaction between your brain and your eyes.

Allow your desire to see clearly to manifest itself in physical restructuring right now.

As you inhale, feel the energy grow in your eyes, and as you exhale, feel the healing which is taking place. Continue with this inhalation of energy, and the exhalation of healing.

And now, simply relax further, let go of the healing exercise, and become even more aware of your breathing. Become one with your breathing, making no conscious effort to breathe.

And allow whatever feelings, memories, insights, or further healing to come to you right now. Let your breathing carry you wherever you need to go, in order to heal on all levels, and to recover your clear vision.

When you are ready, you can slowly start to wake up, to stretch, and perhaps to yawn a couple of invigorating yawns.

Let your eyes open of their own accord, when they want to. Don't anticipate clear vision, simply experience the unique visual state which comes to you as your eyes slowly, effortlessly open and you take in the outside world in a new, refreshing way.

And feel free to go about your day as you wish, remaining aware of your breathing, your eyes, and your desire to see clearly.

With this final healing session of *phase six*, you now have a complete visual recovery programme to work with as you choose. You can see that the various approaches to dealing with myopia offer quite different experiences, which you can choose to suit your temperament.

First we explored simple optic correction through prescription glasses and contact lenses. This is the usual approach to myopia, which corrects the symptom but doesn't deal with the cause.

Secondly we saw that various surgical techniques exist to alter the curvature of the cornea. Corrective lenses have been developed to perform the same flattening function, but all such approaches have thus far proven unsuccessful.

Finally we looked at a new model for myopia, which includes emotional causation as the key principle, and which offers techniques for self-correction and healing.

Although we have considered myopia as a unique problem requiring unique techniques for correction or recovery, we should end this chapter with a reminder that the basic perception and movement exercises presented in Part One of the book are equally important to myopic people. Usually, correcting simple perception habits is the first step in the more advanced work of visual restructuring.

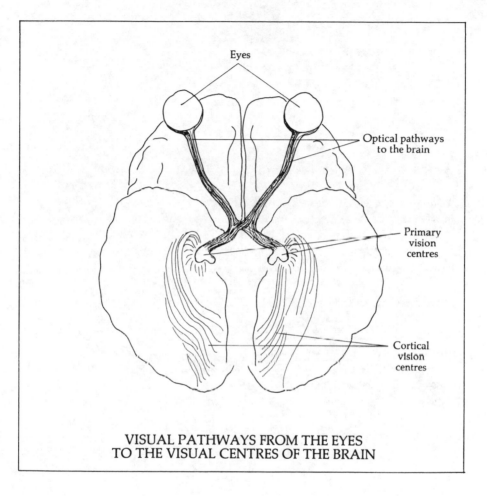

Eyes

Optical pathways
to the brain

Primary
vision
centres

Cortical
vision
centres

**VISUAL PATHWAYS FROM THE EYES
TO THE VISUAL CENTRES OF THE BRAIN**

12 • FAR-SIGHTEDNESS
(Hyperopia and Presbyopia)

Far-sightedness is the opposite of near-sightededness. A person who is far-sighted can usually see clearly in the distance, but has difficulties in focusing on objects which are close to the eyes.

There are two distinct types of far-sightedness. One type, called hyperopia, is usually a childhood affliction related to incorrect shape of the eyes for focusing up-close. As with childhood myopia, the traditional explanation of the cause of hyperopia was genetic: you simply inherited a faulty set of genes which caused the eyeballs to be shaped incorrectly for clear focusing.

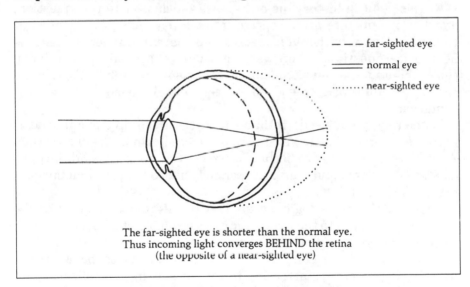

- - - far-sighted eye

====== normal eye

.... near-sighted eye

The far-sighted eye is shorter than the normal eye.
Thus incoming light converges BEHIND the retina
(the opposite of a near-sighted eye)

In fact, it appears that far-sighted children do have eyes which are shaped incorrectly (see illustration). The eyeball is too short from cornea to retina, causing the focal point to land somewhere behind the retina, rather than on the retina. With extra work of the ciliary muscles, the lens can adjust to this condition adequately to bring the distance images into focus on the retina. But the accommodation power of the lens is not strong enough to bring up-close images into

127

focus. Thus the blurred vision and inability to read which many hyperopic children experience.

The standard treatment for hyperopia is optic: reading glasses are required, and for many children, glasses are recommended for both near and also distance vision, to minimize visual stress and resultant headaches.

Curiously, most babies are born with hyperopic eyes, and our first weeks and months of seeing are defined by this inability to focus clearly on near objects. The eyes are not fully developed at birth, and continue to grow and alter their shape for a number of months until sharp focusing is possible.

For this reason, an understanding of hyperopia is possible from the psychological-causation approach, as well as the genetic approach. Research has not yet been completed to determine the accuracy of this new theory, but if you are hyperopic, or if your child has this condition, you can evaluate the logic for yourself: could early childhood traumas inhibit the development of visual functioning and shape? Is there a correlation between negative environmental conditions in infancy and a tendency towards hyperopia?

At this point in history, no one knows the answer to this question, and few eye doctors are receptive to such psychological theories of causation. But as with myopia, we can go one step further and ask the next logical question: if there were a psychological condition in infancy that inhibited the development of the visual system, might it be possible in adulthood, or with youngsters as well, to move beyond this condition?

Concretely, what needs to happen to the hyperopic eye is that it needs to become slightly more elongated, as shown in the illustration. Also, the cornea needs to become *more curved*, so as to bend the light at a greater angle and cause proper focusing on the retinal surface, rather than behind it.

Basically the same logic we applied to internal correction of the myopic eye, applies to the hyperopic eye as well. First of all there needs to be an emotional exploration of remaining contractions which might underline the visual condition. Then there needs to be a precise focusing of the brain's attention to the eyes, using visualizations to encourage an alteration in the physical shape of the eyeball and cornea.

If you are a hyperopic person and wish to explore your potential for such internal alterations, there is a simple cassette programme available which guides you through the two sessions designed to reduce the hyperopic condition. These are experimental programmes which explore your inherent ability to alter your physical functioning. The programmes are in no way dangerous or detrimental to your visual health, and will, in the least, bring you into a closer relationship with your eyes and your healing potential. And the possibility does exist that you do have the ability to recover from your hyperopic condition.

And if you regularly wear hyperopic glasses or contact lenses, you might want to have your prescription reduced one diopter, so that there is room for improvement in your visual system (see page 102). If your glasses do most of the focusing work for you, then your vision will naturally become lazy and inefficient. You should also spend regular hours without wearing your glasses, so that you continue to remain in touch with your natural visual condition, and do not feel totally dependent on your glasses for survival.

Hyperopic children tend to have breathing patterns which inhibit general expression as well. The breathing is usually shallow, high in the chest, and frequently held. This reflects an early childhood condition of apprehension and uncertainty. Even if you do not think you can recover from your visual condition, you should consider whether you have this breath inhibition which limits your emotional and mental functioning, and take steps to recover from this habit.

Specifically, the exercises already described in Part One, which integrate visual movements with smooth rhythmic breathing, are ideal. As soon as you begin to focus on your breathing, you will notice ways in which the full exhalation is blocked, and recurrent times when you hold your breath rather than breathing smoothly through a breath cycle. Simple awareness of your breathing will generate positive alterations. And if you want further guidance in this direction, a complementary text called *Responsive Breathing* is available.

At the moment, there are no surgical interventions which relieve the conditions of hyperopia. Your choice is between wearing glasses and exploring your own healing potential through the programmes mentioned above. There is certainly nothing wrong with simply continuing to wear corrective lenses, but you might surprise yourself at your potential if you begin to consider the possibility of improving your eyesight on your own. Your optometrist will probably laugh at your interest in self-healing, because his experience and training tell him that most people do not recover from hyperopia. But there is no reason for you not being the exception to the rule.

PRESBYOPIA

This second form of far-sightedness is the most common type of visual failure. It is sometimes called 'old-age sight' because it is related to the natural ageing process of the body, and usually develops only after the age of forty. As with hyperopia, presbyopia is an inability to focus clearly on objects which are near to your eyes.

But presbyopia is different from hyperopia in its physical condition.

Whereas hyperopic eyes are distorted through an incorrect shape of the eyeball, the presbyopic eyes actually retain a normal eye shape. The difficulty with presbyopic vision is found in the functioning of the focusing apparatus, specifically the ciliary muscles and the interior lens of the eyes.

As can be seen in the illustration on page 131, the interior lens (as differentiated from the refractive functioning of the cornea) is surrounded by the ciliary muscle. This is a circular muscle which expands its inner diameter when it relaxes, and reduces its diameter when it contracts.

The ciliary muscle is connected to the periphery of the lens by fibres called zonules, which are suspensory ligaments which support the lens in position. When the ciliary muscle is relaxed outward, it pulls on the zonules and thus pulls the lens into a flattened shape, which is necessary for focusing in the distance.

When the ciliary muscle receives orders from the brain to contract, the pressure on the zonules is relieved and the lens assumes its inherent curved shape due to its natural elasticity.

The difficulty called presbyopia develops when the lens begins to lose its natural elasticity, and fails to assume an adequately curved shape when the ciliary muscles contract for up-close vision.

So our question in approaching presbyopia is this: what causes the lens to lose its natural elasticity, gradually reducing the ability of the eye to focus up-close?

The lens consists of remarkable fibres which are both transparent (no pigment or blood supply) and also elastic. These cells are unlike most cells in the body, in that they are not replaced regularly but must function for an entire lifetime. And unfortunately for our visual ability as we grow older, the cells deep within the centre of the lens begin to die as we age, and thus reduce the elastic potential of the lens as a whole.

The reasons for this progressive death of the cells within the lens is not fully understood, but certain factors can be cited. For instance, the lens has no direct blood supply to provide nourishment for its cells, so all nourishment must come indirectly, from the aqueous humour (just as was the case for the cornea). So it seems reasonable to assume that the interior cells, receiving less nutrition than the cells on the surface, will tend to die earlier. They are also the oldest cells of the lens, and thus might suffer from the realities of old age as does the rest of the body.

So in considering preventative programmes for postponing presbyopia, circulation and diet should play a vital role in helping to maintain optimum health of the cells within the lens.

Another factor which is often forgotten in the consideration of presbyopia, is the health and vitality of the ciliary muscle surrounding

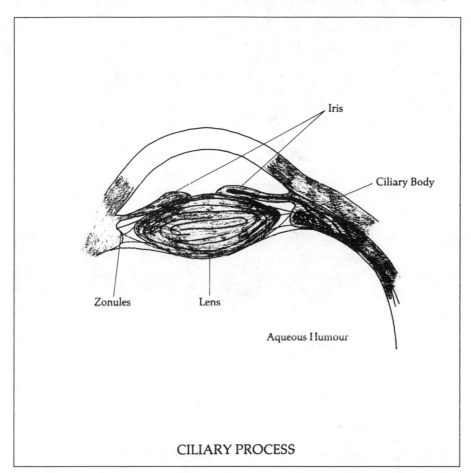

Iris

Ciliary Body

Zonules

Lens

Aqueous Humour

CILIARY PROCESS

and controlling the shape of the lens. Like all muscles in our bodies, this muscle can be in good shape or in poor shape. And like the rest of our body, the ciliary muscle can age relatively early in life, or remain strong and vital to a very old age.

The process of ageing certainly has its genetic components, but we know from everyday experience that our basic attitudes towards life determine much of our vitality and sense of youthfulness. Some people appear to be rigid and ageing at 40, whereas others approach 80 with zest, physical agility, and strength.

Likewise, there are people who must use reading glasses at the age of 35, and there are others who reach the age of 70 and are still able to read the evening paper without glasses. When an optometrist says that you will need reading glasses after the age of 40, he is assuming that you fit the normal stereotype for health in our present civilization. Perhaps you do. But on the other hand, perhaps you will remain in that minority that retains up-close focusing ability to a much older age.

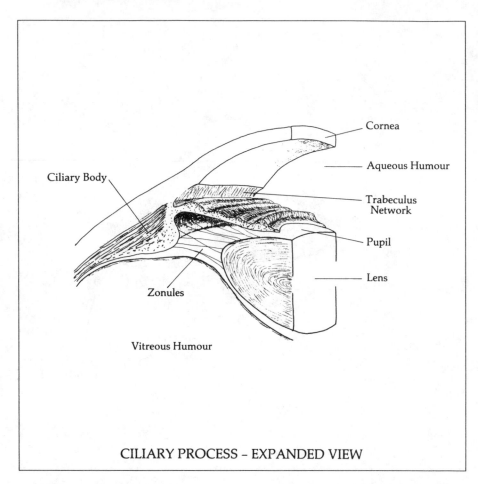

CILIARY PROCESS – EXPANDED VIEW

We do exercises and try to maintain a healthy diet for the rest of our body. Why don't we care for our eyes as well? Why is it that we have ignored practical routines for vision health, when we daily spend time with our dental health?

Unfortunately, optometrists during their professional training are usually instructed that it is best to prepare their patients for the eventual development of presbyopia. Thus, we are told that it is natural to lose our clear vision after the age of 40, and that we should anticipate this development. We are programmed to believe that our eyes will fail us. What effect does this programming have on our visual vitality?

In working with presbyopic clients, I have seen time and again that temporary periods of complete up-close focusing occur when the person is in a relaxed, expansive, unconstricted state of mind. Presbyopia is an extremely variable condition. When a client is locked into a habitual self-concept of fatigue, time pressure, and lost vitality, presbyopia prevails. When the self-image is set aside and the person feels full of vitality, free of emotional restrictions, and joyful, visual functioning returns to the potential of earlier years.

So in dealing with presbyopia, we need to see that we are not dealing with a simple physiological development, static and not reversible. We are dealing with a general mind-state which manifests itself in the physical body. Most doctors will agree with the determining factor of attitude in physical health. To a large degree, we do create our illnesses, our infirmities, and certainly our premature ageing syndromes.

And on the other hand, we have the personal choice of maintaining a healthy, vital attitude towards life, and of consciously helping our eyes to remain youthful many years past 40.

POSTPONING PRESBYOPIA

From the age of 20 we can work towards postponing the final ageing cycle of our eyes, and of the rest of our body as well. We can get adequate exercise, we can eat well-balanced diets, and we can do the special vision exercises which will be discussed in a moment.

But deeper that these specific approaches to remaining healthy is a new view of health which will hopefully become a major determinant in future programmes. As outlined by doctors such as Larry Dossey in his book *Space, Time and Medicine*, our basic perception of time itself seems to aggravate the ageing process. We can perceive the flow of time in many different ways. But our modern culture presses us into experiencing time as a fleeting, pressurized movement. We are forced from early childhood to be always rushing to school, rushing to work, always racing against the clock.

The result is a general tension and a feeling that time is slipping away from us. Also, we are conditioned to see our lives not as expansive, present-oriented experiences, but as a certain, all-too-rapid march towards the grave. We are a culture which spends so much time worrying about the future, that we barely take time to enjoy the present. And this stress certainly generates an acceleration in the ageing process. We work and hurry so much that all we can look forward to is retirement and a few final years of peace before we enter the old people's home and die.

So one of the best ways of postponing presbyopia is to begin to shift our perspective on time to a more relaxed, present-oriented experience. Almost every job in our culture requires us to look up-close most of the time. So when we take a break, we should look into the distance. And for general circulation health, we should take a deep breath regularly, stretch, and allow our bodies to recover from the tensions of a time-pressurized civilization.

An interesting theory of presbyopia sheds further light on the condition. Traditionally, we did much less up-close work than we do now. Certainly, little children weren't forced to attend schools and constantly look up-close at books for hours on end as they do nowadays. The eyes were much freer, and were in the relaxed, distance-viewing state much of the time.

So perhaps around the age of 40 a deep part of us simply gets tired of forcing the eyes to do so much up-close focusing. Perhaps at a deeper psychological level, we revolt against the lifetime of pressurized visual work, and start to blur all the up-close work out of our lives. Presbyopia would then be a reaction, not a natural process.

In fact, most presbyopia clients I have worked with agree, after honest introspection, that they are definitely tired of the tensions associated with up-close looking. At some level, they would like to let go of the pressures which have usually been related to reading, operating machinery, etc.

Certainly this factor is at least one dimension of the development of presbyopia.

Wilhelm Reich, one of the pioneers of modern psychology, made a further comment on presbyopia. He suggested that we begin to lose our ability to look up-close at the same time that we begin to age physically, and that it is our denial to see the ageing process in our own body that leads to presbyopia. If we blur the first few feet in front of us into non-existence, then we can avoid the direct experience of our ageing.

Such psychological explanations do not fully explain conditions such as presbyopia, because certainly, the natural ageing process will have its effects on vision as well as on other parts of the body. But there seems to be an important grain of truth in such observations. If we do not accept our coming death through the ageing process, we will naturally want to avoid seeing any evidence of our ageing.

The question of import is: to what extent do you accept the natural ageing process of your own body? Are you able to accept your imminent death? And can you slow down from the hectic pace of modern life and allow your eyes to relax and enjoy the present visual experience around you?

Meditating regularly on such questions can provide the necessary groundwork for the success of the exercises which follow.

OPTOMETRIC TREATMENT OF PRESBYOPIA

Optometrists are almost always very nice people. They want you to be comfortable with your reading glasses , so that your eyes won't have to work hard at all in order to see up-close. So it is common practice to prescribe glasses which are one diopter too strong for your present visual needs. This gives you what they call a 'comfort zone', so that the ciliary muscles won't have to work to focus up-close.

On one hand, this is very helpful. But from another point of view, over-prescribing for presbyopia will generate a rapid deterioration in ciliary-muscle functioning, so that your visual condition will be reduced more rapidly than normally. The ciliary muscle is like any other muscle. If you don't use it, its strength will fade away.

So if you find that you do need glasses for reading, or if you already wear such glasses for up-close work, please remember your ciliary muscles, and give them plenty of exercise. When you go to get new glasses, make sure they are not too strong. And do as much of your visual work as you can without the help of glasses. Keep your eyes working!

The same applies to your body in general. Walk instead of taking the car, carry your groceries to give your muscles a good workout, and instead of avoiding physical exertion, seek it, enjoy the rush of expanded breathing that comes with exercising, and let your body stay strong and flexible well into old age.

I am often asked about bi-focals. People who need glasses to read up-close often get bi-focals which have clear glass in the top portion of the frame, and reading lenses in the lower portion of the glasses. This is done for comfort, so that you don't have to reach for your glasses to see something up-close.

From a practical point of view, bi-focals make sense. But from a deeper point of view, beware of them. As mentioned earlier, studies have indicated that looking at the world through glass reduces your emotional response to the world around you. You are putting a barrier of glass between you and your friends. Everyone knows that it is more difficult to look into the eyes of a person wearing glasses than a person without glasses. Perhaps the ritual of reaching for your glasses to see up-close is worth the freedom you maintain when looking in the distance. Your choice, but be sure you consider all the alternatives.

One further recommendation. When you find that you need a new pair of glasses because your eyes get tired reading at night, keep your old pair also. When you are alert and your eyes are not tired, wear the old, weaker glasses. Only wear the stronger ones when your eyes are tired. Presbyopia is definitely a factor of ciliary muscle fatigue, and you should only wear stronger lenses when the muscles are especially tired.

SPECIFIC PRESBYOPIA EXERCISES

I developed the following exercise programme several years ago for the

American Airline Pilots Association. It offers a quick five-minute routine which you can do regularly, both to postpone the onset of presbyopia, and to reduce its condition if you already have difficulty in focusing up-close.

Rapid Focal Shifting

This exercise, modified from the traditional Bates 'whipping' exercise, provides the ciliary muscles with an especially vigorous physical work-out, which should always be followed by six breath cycles of the 'palming' relaxation exercise described before.

Cover your *left* eye with your *right* hand allowing your left eye to remain open under the cupped palm.

Move your *left* hand, palm towards your face, close to your *right* eye, and then move it out away from that eye as you watch it closely, noting the details of the lines in your palm. Move your hand away to arm's length in front of you, and then move the hand towards the eye again until it goes out of focus.

Inhale for one cycle, then exhale for the next, for perhaps ten cycles. Palm with both eyes covered, for six breaths. Then reverse the process and exercise the ciliary muscle in the left eye, and palm afterwards. Be sure to remain aware of your breathing and the feeling in your eyes.

Neck and Scalp Relaxation

Chronic tension in the neck and scalp seems to be a factor in presbyopic eyestrain, linked with ciliary tensions. You can regularly reduce this tension by the following exercise.

Stand up preferably, and slowly begin shaking your head from one side to the other. Make sure to breathe through your mouth as you do this, to relax the tensions in the jaw and tongue. Make a soft 'aaahhh' sound as you move your head from side to side, rotating gently from the neck.

As you do this swinging of the head, raise and lower your head slowly, so as to loosen all the different muscles in the neck.

Then slowly bend over forwards towards the ground, your arms relaxed, your breathing full through the mouth, with your knees slightly bent. Touch the floor with your hands, and slowly move the head back and forth again, allowing the blood to flow into your head to revitalize your eyes. Make soft sounds as you swing your head, and allow your neck muscles to relax further.

Then very slowly, stand up, feeling your vertebra straightening upwards one at a time, until your head finally comes upright.

Gently pound on your head for further loosening up of the

extraocular muscles and to encourage maximum circulation in the eye themselves. Continue making a soft 'aaahhhhh' sound as you pound. Lower your head and pound on the neck too!

VISUALIZATION SESSION

As with myopia, the power of your brain to bring about changes in the structures of your eyes with presbyopia can be tapped through visualization exercises. This is an experimental technique, but one which shows great promise. If you can send orders to the lens, ciliary muscles, and cornea to slightly alter their shape and functioning so as to encourage up-close focusing, you can begin to take the health of your eyes into your own hands.

The interaction of our consciousness with our physical bodies is still an uncharted dimension of human existence. In doing this visualization session, you are exploring your ability to heal yourself. For many of us, it is quite an amazing experience to focus our attention directly on our eyes, to see how they actually feel, and to direct healing attention to them. Play with this visualization lightly, and simply experience its validity for your own eyes.

Sit or lie down comfortably, where you can be at peace for about ten or fifteen minutes. Take off your shoes if they are tight, and allow yourself to relax. Close your eyes and focus on the sensation of the air going in and out through your nose with each breath. Watch your breathing, while making absolutely no effort to breathe. Just passively observe how your present breathing reflects your general state of mind and body.

Allow your awareness to expand to include your entire head, so that you are conscious of the space inside your skull. Breathe into this space, and allow it to relax and expand.

Now, while still aware of your breathing, expand your awareness to include your entire body at once, without effort. Simply be aware of yourself as a whole being, present in space, and breathing.

Bring your attention gently to your heart. Be aware of it beating inside your chest. Allow yourself to feel the life pulsating inside you. Notice the sensation which comes to you when you become aware of your heart, and your breathing, at the same time. Allow this feeling to expand, and enjoy the simple experience of being alive right now, your mind quiet, your breathing calm, your heart strong and expansive.

Now allow your attention to expand to include your throat. Feel this area relaxing, your tongue relaxing, your jaw relaxing, so that your breathing becomes more even, softer, effortless through your vocal chords.

Bring your awareness up to your eyes themselves now, without effort.

Simply be aware of the eyes as they rest in your head, and notice what sensations you feel coming from them to your consciousness.

Visualize the presence of your ciliary muscle surrounding the lens in each eye. Encourage this muscle to relax.

Now imagine that you are looking at something that is very close to your face, your own hand perhaps, or the face of a friend. Feel your ciliary muscles contracting, and your lens springing into its more rounded shape.

Experience an effortless focusing on this close focus. Breathe in a relaxed way, exhaling completely, as you imagine looking up close with no strain at all.

Now look off into the distance in your imagination, and allow the ciliary muscles to relax.

Again imagine looking very close to something or someone, and without effort seeing what you are looking at in complete clear focus. Breathe and enjoy this effortless focusing.

And now just relax the eyes and let go of the visualization. Breathe, be aware of your body.

Return your focus to your eyes. Focus on your lens in each eye, the actual presence of this living bundle of cells. Encourage an increased health and vitality of these cells, with oxygen and nutrition flowing inward to the centre of the lens, bringing increased vitality to the cells.

Imagine the lens becoming more elastic, more flexible, able to flex into its round natural posture for up-close seeing. And imagine your ciliary muscles feeling vital, in top shape, eager to contract so that the lens can focus up-close whenever such focusing is needed in the future.

And now just relax, sigh a deep sigh through the mouth on your next exhalation, and enjoy the feeling of relaxation and vitality in your eyes.

You can stay in this relaxed state for as long as you wish, and when you want to return to your normal activities, you can open your eyes, stretch and yawn, and carry on with your day.

This is the basic presbyopia programme, and you can do it once a week of as often as three times a day, depending on your need and motivation.

If simple eye-strain is a problem for you, remember that the palming exercise presented earlier, in conjunction with a conscious focus on your breathing, will quickly relax the muscles of the eyes and relieve eye-strain in most cases. If you continue to have tensions in the eyes, the full-body relaxation session in Part One is recommended (see pages 57-58).

13 · CATARACTS
('Old Age Blindness')

Complementary to our discussion of presbyopia is a consideration of the condition called cataracts, because both conditions are primarily focused on the lens inside the eye, and both are usually associated with ageing.

A cataract is any clouding of the crystalline lens so that the passage of light through the lens is interfered with. Although usually a problem of old age, people of all ages can develop cataracts, and even newborn babies sometimes have cataract clouding in the lens. Such diverse conditions as measles, diabetes, reaction to drugs, eye injuries, and alterations in body metabolism are associated with the development of cataracts.

As with so many other visual conditions, there is still no scientific explanation for the development of cataracts, and throughout the literature on the subject we encounter such statements as 'no one really understands fully what causes the lens to turn cloudy.'[1] In fact, the basic causation models in most illnesses are currently under question, as the impact of Einsteinian relativity and quantum mechanics data put into doubt the models of molecular biophysics. All we can point to currently is the rising evidence that health and disease are factors of the individual in relationship to the environment. Our attitudes, diet, exercise, sense of time, and emotional health seem as important as our genetic and biological dimensions in remaining healthy, Cataract development certainly fits into this understanding also.

But regardless of the causes of cataracts, thay are a primary source of visual failure. Over 400,000 cataract extractions are performed through eye surgery each year in the United States alone, and it is estimated that over 10 million individuals become visually disabled in the United States each year because of cataract.[2] Fifteen per cent of the population between the ages of 52 and 85 have cataracts which noticeably reduce their visual potential.

[1]*Eyewise*, page 46
[2]L. V. Mosby, *Ophthalmology Principles and Concepts*, page 377 (St Louis, 1961).

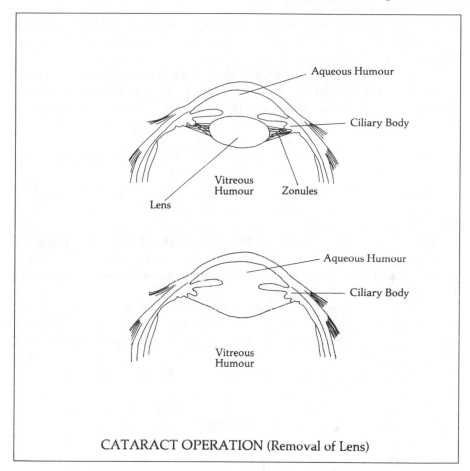

Aqueous Humour

Ciliary Body

Vitreous
Humour   Zonules

Lens

Aqueous Humour

Ciliary Body

Vitreous
Humour

CATARACT OPERATION (Removal of Lens)

The symptoms of cataract development are a decrease in visual acuity which is not associated with pain or inflammation of the eye. Some people experience this loss of clear vision as a film or cloud over the eye, others complain of general blurriness. Certain types of cataracts also cause exaggerated glare from oncoming headlights of cars.

In all cases, the lens itself is developing parts which are no longer transparent. Sometimes this development takes place in the centre of the lens. At other times the outer portions of the lens are affected first.

Cataracts can take years to develop, or can develop very rapidly in a matter of weeks or months. They can develop in both eyes, or at first just in one eye. But regardless of the pace and mode of development, the resultant loss of clear vision is very disturbing to the sufferer, and anxiety and confusion make matters worse.

If you suspect that your vision is failing, for any reason, it is always a good idea to have your eyes inspected by an eye doctor. With cataracts, doctors can simply inspect the lens through various methods which are quick and painless, and let you know the actual developments inside your eyes.

Except for surgical removal, there are presently no accepted treatments for cataracts. The approach of the medical community is simply to allow the cataract to 'ripen', to get extremely cloudy, and then to cut the lens out of the eye so that it no longer blocks the light coming through the eye to the retina.

Interestingly, we find such comments in medical books related to cataracts. 'No treatment will restore the denatured protein of the cataractous lens to its original transparent state. *However, lens vacuoles may at times disappear spontaneously and give rise to an improvement in vision.*'[3]

This indicates that at times, the eyes somehow act to correct the poor state of health of the lens. Doctors don't know how to affect this reversal in cataract development, but some individuals spontaneously heal themselves.

As with presbyopia, prevention is the best approach to cataract development, and we apply the same basic principles. The health of the lens cells is dependent upon proper nutrition, adequate circulation of the blood, adequate oxygenation, and probably regular activity of the lens (accommodation, or focusing near and far regularly without the hindrance of reading glasses).

Basic exercise routines for visual health have been presented fully in Part One, and I refer you to those chapters for guidance.

SURGICAL INTERVENTION

The removal of a cataract lens is one of the safest and most common surgical procedures performed by doctors each day throughout the world. There are two basic approaches to this surgery. Traditionally, a rather large incision is made around the edge of the cornea, and the lens is carefully extracted. The operation takes about an hour, and usually you can leave the hospital after a day or two of recovery. Several months are required for complete healing of the eye however, and caution must be taken against pushing or straining during this time.

The second approach to cataract removal, usually performed only on those under 45, is called phakoemulsification, and involves pulverizing the lens before removing it from the eye. This is done with a tiny vibrating device which works like a microscopic jackhammer, pounding away 40,000 times a second on the lens and breaking it into tiny pieces. These pieces are then suctioned out of the eye.

[3] L.V. Mosby, *Opthalmology*, page 382 (my italics).

Because the incision needed for this type of cataract removal is only one-tenth of an inch, the surgery trauma to the eye is greatly reduced, and the patient can recover much faster from the operation, usually in two or three weeks.

For complex physiological reasons, this operation does not work well with people over 60 years of age, but is especially applicable to people under 40. Your physician can advise you as to which approach would be preferable in your particular case.

Once you have recovered from the surgery, the second half of the task remains. You have eliminated the cloudy lens which obstructed your vision. But in doing so, you have lost the focusing element which fine-tunes the image entering the eye so that it lands in focus on the retina. After a cataract operation, the world is a vague blur. Beyond a foot or two, you can't even distinguish your own hand.

The solution to this condition must rest with corrective lenses. These are either glasses or contact lenses, which do the general work of the lens. Obviously, external lenses will not be able to change their shape to fine-focus like the crystalline lens could, but vision will be greatly improved, so that you can drive a car for instance. When compared with the progressive blindness which cataracts develop, this partial recovery of clear functional vision is a blessing.

With younger people, contact lenses are usually advised, because the heavy thick glass required for clear vision after cataract surgery causes considerable distortion in image size and peripheral vision with normal glasses. But with older people, using contact lenses is very often difficult, due to eye sensitivity, insufficient tear flow, and the difficulty of regularly putting the lenses in and out of the eyes. New types of lens material have considerably reduced the 'coke bottle' reputation of traditional cataract lenses.

There is a third approach to correcting visual acuity after a cataract extraction. This is to implant an artificial plastic lens into the eye, to replace the natural one which has been removed. This is a procedure which has interested eye surgeons for decades, but it still remains complicated and uncertain as to long-term results.

The implantation of an artificial lens is usually recommended only for people who have lost one lens, but retain a healthy lens in the other eye. Because corrective lenses do not completely match image size with that of the natural lens, the brain receives two different-sized images, which generates serious confusion. Implantation of an artificial 'intraocular' lens overcomes this difficulty.

But complications exist, making this implantation less than ideal with existing technological expertise. For instance, no long-term tests have been made on permanent success for the implantation, and the artificial lenses can slip from position inside the eye, causing trauma and possibly damage to the retina or cornea. Infection is always a possibility, because the plastic lens generates chronic irritation inside the eye. And there is the possibility that the material of the artificial lens might disintegrate within the eye after a certain time and cause blindness.

For these reasons, intraocular lens implantation is now generally reserved only for elderly patients with a cataract in only one eye. Future improvements in the implantation approach will possibly expand this range to include others as well.

ALTERNATIVE APPROACHES TO CATARACT TREATMENT

Until recently, doctors have scoffed at the idea that comeone could alter his or her physical condition through the conscious activity of the mind. The body has traditionally been seen as a complex cellular machine which is not responsive to the parallel world of our consciousness.

But with the advent of the new physics and the deeply penetrating reverberations of the theories of relativity and quantum mechanics, our scientific understanding of the mind/body duality has undergone a radical shift. Even such renowned scholarly groups as the American Association for the Advancement of Science have held conferences on such themes as 'The Role of Consciousness in the Physical World', with conclusions generally running on the lines of the following:

> The new view of consciousness asserts unabashedly that conscious mental activity exerts measureable effects on the physical world – a world which includes human bodies, organs, tissues, and cells. Mind becomes a legitimate factor in the unfolding of health and disease.[4]

Thus, in considering whether we do have any ability to bring about a conscious alteration of our cellular functioning, the answer from the scientific point of view seems to be, more and more definitely, 'Yes!'.

The practical task at hand, then, is the development of a programme which will successfully focus your conscious attention on your lens itself. Once this focusing has been attained, the proper images and motivational attitude will be necessary in order to have the desired effect in your lens tissue.

Such a programme is certainly experimental. As with the myopia programme presented already, and the glaucoma programme coming in a later chapter, this cataract reversal programme is a safe, enjoyable exploration of your personal potential for reversing a negative

[4]L. Dossey, *Space, Time, and Medicine*, page 209.

144

condition in your body, through conscious focusing of your brainpower on that region.

Some people develop cataracts, but the majority of us do not. Are those of us who develop cloudy lenses simply victims of fate and biology, of genetic predisposition and statistical body failure syndromes? How do you feel about your responsibility in generating a cataract, if you have one? Are you in charge of your body, or is your body some separate mechanism from your consciousness, operating without any influence of your deeper feelings and habits?

The premise of this alternative cataract reversal programme is that we are all responsible for our own health. This directly implies that our lifelong habits of negative mental patterns, constricted emotional patterns, and dietary and exercise routines, all contribute to our development of illness at some point in our lives. Do you feel that this is true in your particular case?

Assuming responsibility for the development of cataracts is not the same as feeling guilty, by the way. To assume responsibility for your cellular health is simply to accept what appears to be a physiological reality. And only if you accept this reality and act within its natural laws, can you consciously choose to improve your cellular health.

What we need to do in this programme, and in any healing programme which is internally directed, is to establish a line of communication between the brain (your consciousness) and the individual cells needing help and correction.

Cells are individual beings in their own right, as shown by recent biochemical research. The idea of cellular intelligence is just beginning to emerge, but in fact, each cell in your body is a complete living unit. Each cell breathes, consumes nourishment, excretes waste, and has a 'brain' called the nucleus. Within the nucleus are some forty-six chromosomes, each of which houses a vast number of genes. It is the genes which would appear to be the heart of the intelligence of a cell.

And therefore it is with these genes that the brain must communicate, and in fact is communicating all the time. With each surge of emotion you feel, for instance, an energy flow radiates throughout your body, influencing the functioning and health of your cells.

If a person approaching the last phase of life on planet Earth is regularly thinking and feeling such thoughts as 'life is horrible, painful, I don't want to face it anymore, I'm growing old and feel so tired of life', these thoughts and the accompanying emotions radiate throughout the body. And as I suggested in discussing childhood myopia, there is a good possibility that the cells in the eyes respond to this continual state of consciousness with biochemical changes which reflect the mental state.

Put simply, at some level, people who develop cataracts might be emotionally tired of facing life out there. Even if the feeling is unconscious, it still radiates and affects the body on several different planes.

So a change in attitude seems required in order for a change in physical health to really occur. This is an observation made by generations of doctors regarding why some people recover from an illness, and others die from the same condition. Our will to live, our basic vibratory state, directly influences the functioning of our organism.

So to begin with, you might want to consider how you feel about looking at the outside world. Even though you want to see clearly out of the fear of being blind, even though you need to see clearly to function effectively and survive on your own – do you really *desire* to see clearly? What is your emotional feeling towards seeing the present world and its daily changes? Are you really wanting to blur away the outside world?

An interesting statistic about elderly people with cataracts is that the majority of them prefer not to have the cataract-extraction operation which would restore their sight. They choose instead to go blind. What does this mean? Certainly some of them are frightened of the operation and avoid it. And some of them have spiritual reasons for accepting their natural progression towards death. Bur probably the pervading feeling is that they simply don't want to see anymore. They prefer to regress into their inner worlds of memories, to replay the inner visual films of better times in the past. Senility, like cataract development, appears to be at least partly the direct result of an unconscious (or even conscious) choice to let go of the present world, and to withdraw into the inner realms of memory and spiritual preparation for death.

I hope it is clear that I am not judging this decision to withdraw. Death is the final stage of life for all of us, and at some point, we do need to turn inward and beyond, to focus away from the material world around us and return to our deeper centre.

This programme for cataract reversal is intended for those of you who, perhaps inadvertently, unconsciously allowed habitual thought patterns to undermine your visual health, and who want to reverse this development so that, at least for the next phase of your life, you continue to see clearly and to keep your health vibrant and linked with the flow of events around you.

Also, if you are reading this chapter because you have a loved one who is developing cataracts, and you want to know how you can be of help, an honest discussion of this chapter would be perhaps the best approach. Often, the development of cataracts indicates the beginnings of honesty about ageing and death in general within families, and this is a very healthy development. To ask a person with cataracts how he or she really feels about ageing and death is usually to invite a deep discussion which otherwise might not happen. And it is important, as an act of love, to encourage such discussions, rather than leaving the cataract patient alone with the progressive visual failure.

So honesty, discussion, reflection and emotional expression are all part of a general approach to cataract development and possible reversal. Discussion involves mysterious interaction, because we find ourselves thinking and talking about feelings and ideas which otherwise do not rise to the surface and become conscious. If we approach cataract development as a reflection of a deeper progression, rather than just an isolated accident of the body, we can delve into the depths of our being. This is the positive aspect of cataract development – it can open doors to communication, reflection, and the activation of one's latent healing potential.

And it is never too late to begin this exploration of our hidden reserves.

VISUALIZATION OF CATARACT REVERSAL

The procedure for this healing session is similar to that with presbyopia as given in the last chapter. The aim is to learn to direct your consciousness to your eyes, and to focus your desire to heal on this region of your body. The basic visualization and healing session is presented below, and you can obtain the expanded half-hour cassette programme if you want a voice to guide you through the process. You will want to do this session at least three times a week, in order to develop your ability to focus your healing attention on the cells in your lens.

This session is also a valuable preventative programme in combination with the general health and visual performance exercises in Part One. Regardless of your age, you can go through this relaxing half-hour and enjoy the feeling of directly turning your love and attention to the health of your eyes. For best results do this regularly, perhaps once a week.

Find a quiet place to sit or lie down, where you can be undisturbed for perhaps twenty minutes to half an hour. Be sure to wear loose clothing when possible, for ease of breathing.

Turn your focus to your breathing, with your eyes closed. Feel the air going in and out of your nose, the actual sensation of the flow of air.

Allow this awareness to expand to include your whole head at once, while you remain aware of your breathing, and allow it to expand and relax step by step.

Effortlessly, allow your awareness to expand to include your whole body at once, as you remain aware of your breathing through your nose. Feel the presence of your body in the room, from the tip of your toes to the top of your head.

Now allow your awareness to begin to focus especially on your eyes. Do this gently, without force, simply encouraging your consciousness to turn its attention the actual presence of your eyes in your head.

Feel if they are tense or relaxed, and with every breath, encourage further relaxation. Move the eyes gently as if looking in different directions for a moment, to become more conscious of their presence. Then relax and simply hold your attention to your eyes as you breathe.

Focus your attention on the outer surface of the eyes, the cornea, for a moment. Actually be aware of this surface under your closed lids. Raise a hand up to each eye and lightly touch this surface through your closed lids, to bring tactile awareness more strongly to your eyes.

Now allow your awareness to move a step within your eyes themselves, so that your awareness is directed to the lens within each eye. Feel the presence of the lens. Breathe into this awareness and allow it to expand, so that all of your attention is consciously focused on the millions of cells which make up each lens.

Allow a flow of love and acceptance to move effortlessly up through your body, and out to your eyes and the lenses. Focus this flow to the eye which needs the most attention and healing.

Now allow yourself to experience the millions of intelligent cells which make up your lenses. Feel their openness to whatever communication you now send to them. And allow your desire to see clearly to flow to these cells, so that they receive clearly your desire and request for a reversal of the conditions causing your cataract.

Continue to allow this flow of loving attention and energy to move up through your body, gaining specific instructions from your brain regarding cellular vitality and functioning, and then flowing out to the cells in your lenses.

Enjoy this effortless flow. Feel how your entire body begins to feel more alive, vibrant, healthy.

Breathe into the process and continue to send the healing energy and information to your lenses, with the wisdom of the brain directing the needed changes towards health.

And allow whatever emotions and insights that might be rising to the surface to become conscious now.

Be open to any feelings which might be associated with your cataract condition. Let these feelings come out. There can be tears, anger, joy, sadness, hope, whatever feelings are there, allow them to come out now.

And if there are thoughts which rise up from your deeper consciousness, meditate on these insights, allow them to bring about their own changes which are needed for further health and vitality.

And when you are ready, you can end this session, return to your wakeful state, stretch, yawn, and go on about your day with a revitalized feeling in your eyes and body!

14 · THE GLAUCOMAS
(Inner Eye Pressure)

The term Glaucoma carries with it an aura both of mystery and anxiety. Glaucoma is a devious condition, in that no noticeable symptoms develop until after damage has actually begun to occur in the visual system. The only early detection method is a regular yearly check-up with the eye doctor, who can perform simple tests to determine if glaucoma is or is not developing.

As we have already seen briefly, the interior of the eye is filled primarily with liquid. There are two main chambers inside the eye, the frontal chamber which is filled with aqueous humour, and the back chamber which is filled with a more permanent jelly called vitreous humour.

Glaucoma is a condition which develops in the frontal, aqueous chamber, and which then affects the entire eye in that it increases the overall pressure inside the eye.

There are two alternative understandings of the cause and treatment of glaucoma. First we will consider the traditional medical model of this condition, and then we shall expand the discussion to explore a more holistic understanding, and present a new method of treatment. These two approaches are not mutually exclusive. Actually, the newer approach builds upon the firm base of medical science, and looks one step further into the causal factors of the condition. With both points of view in place, we should gain a stereoscopic perspective on the problem, and have a clear notion of how to proceed.

As with all other parts of the body, the eye must maintain an optimum balance between the outside world and the interior realms. With glaucoma, we find the development of a crucial imbalance. The interior pressure of the eye begins to increase, generating numerous complications for the functioning and health of the organ.

There are two chief characters in this story. First of all, there is the ciliary body which produces aqueous humour. Part of the ciliary body, as we have discussed, surrounds the lens and is responsible for altering the shape of the lens for accommodation. But a large portion of the ciliary body has quite a different function in the eye. It receives a rich supply of blood, and transforms this blood into a clear liquid called the aqueous humour.

This clear liquid enters the frontal chamber of the eye, and provides essential nutrients for both the crystalline lens and the cornea. This liquid flows down through the frontal chamber, makes its exchange with the lens and cornea, and then is filtered out of the eye through a complex mesh network which returns the liquid to the bloodstream for its return to the lungs and heart.

A pre-glaucoma condition develops when the creation of aqueous humour becomes greater than the outflow of the liquid. The pressure thus increases in the eye, and the damage caused by this increased pressure is called glaucoma.

As with any pressurized container, the eye will tend to break down, or 'blow out', at its weakest point, when the pressure becomes too great. In the case of the eye, this point is where the retina enters the optic nerve passageway on its trip to the brain. Over a million individual fibres, each connected with a retinal photo-receptor, pass through the entry into the optic nerve. And for some reason, it is here that damage first occurs in glaucoma.

In simple terms, the fibres begin to break as the interior pressure of the eye increases. This is a permanent damage, resulting in the direct loss of neural communication between the retina and the visual centres of the brain. So if glaucoma continues without control and a reduction in the aqueous pressure, more and more of the optic nerve is severed, and vision begins to be reduced.

At first, this breakage of retinal fibres affects only the peripheral vision of the eye, so that you can still see quite clearly, but with a reduced-size image. Finally, the central, foveal fibres break down also under the pressure, and complete and permanent loss of vision in that eye is experienced,

Traditionally, the aim of medical treatment of glaucoma has been to detect an increase in pressure of the eye as soon as possible, and to use drugs to control the pressure so that no more damage will be done to the optic nerve. If the condition is detected soon enough, lifetime drug therapy can control glaucoma and preserve the vision intact.

This means that each of us should have our eyes periodically checked, to determine whether eye pressure is becoming too high.

There are drugs which help to increase the flow of aqueous humour out of the eye, and also drugs which serve to reduce the amount of aqueous humour being produced by the ciliary body. Either or both treatments are the standard control for glaucoma.

If these treatments do not succeed in reducing the pressure to a safe level, then surgery is recommended. In most cases, the operation involves cleaning out the drainage system of the aqueous humour,

151

either through opening channels for the liquid to flow through, or through implanting actual pipes to carry the liquid away.

These operations are about 80 per cent successful, but can result in the development of cataracts, in infection which can blind the eye, and in too great a loss of pressure so that the eye does not see clearly.

In a small percentage of glaucoma cases (closed angle glaucoma), surgery is required, because the iris has slipped forward and totally blocks the outflow of aqueous humour. But in most cases, doctors prefer to treat the condition with drugs and use surgery only as a final effort to preserve the vision in the eye.

The commonest type of glaucoma is called 'open angle glaucoma', because the angle between the iris and the cornea remains open, and a more subtle blockage of the actual filter system causes the increased pressure. This glaucoma, called 'acute glaucoma' also, makes up about 99 per cent of all glaucoma cases, and thus deserves our central focus of attention.

The two key words in the outflow mechanism of the aqueous humour are the Canal of Schlemm, which is the main pipeline carrying the humour to the bloodstream, and the trabecular meshwork, the fine filter which allows the liquid to seep slowly down into the Canal of Schlemm.

The Canal of Schlemm, as seen in the illustration, surrounds the anterior chamber, and is usually not a causal factor in the reduction of outflow of aqueous humour. The real mystery surrounds the progressive failure of the trabecular meshwork to pass aqueous humour to the Canal of Schlemm.

Such drugs as pilocarpine and echotheophate iodide are prescribed when eye pressure is determined to be too high (there is no set pressure regarded as the critical pressure beyond which treatment is called for, but normally a pressure of over 22 mm Hg generates concern). These drugs serve to increase the permeability of the trabecular meshwork, thus reducing pressure. The proper dosage requires repeated trial-and-error experiments until an equilibrium is maintained.

Ephinephrine and eserine drops serve the opposite purpose, that of reducing the secretion of aqueous humour by the ciliary body. Both treatments may be used at the same time.

The actual eye pressure is tested with the use of a tonometer which directly tests the pressure needed to indent the outer surface of the cornea. The test is painless, quick, and in no way dangerous to undergo once a year or every two years. Doctors recommend this test, and others, for everyone.

Glaucoma is primarily associated with the ageing process. Approximately 2 per cent of the population are expected to develop the condition during their lifetime. Untreated glaucoma is a serious cause of blindness in the population, and prevention through testing and drug treatment is the primary approach of the medical establishment.

Actually, no one knows the cause of the dysfunction of the trabecular meshwork. In closed angle glaucoma there seems to be a definite correlation between emotional trauma and slippage of the iris to close off the drainage passageway. But in the primary open-angle glaucoma, causality remains a mystery.

So from a medical point of view, have your eyes checked regularly for ocular pressure, and if you are diagnosed as having too high a pressure, take your eye drops regularly for the rest of your life.

THE ALTERNATIVE APPROACH

We now take a step back from the medical model, and consider the human being as a whole. What does it mean that the eye pressure is increasing? If we put aside the concept that we are pure victims of the ravages of disease, and consider the possibility that we in fact generate our physical ailments why would this condition develop?

The emotional causation theme has long been popular with glaucoma patients, and certain ophthalmologists as well.

A traditionalist text on glaucoma states:

There seems to be a great tendency among patients to wonder whether nervousness or anxiety has an adverse influence on their glaucoma. Some ophthalmologists are convinced that such is the case. However, the evidence looks quite inconclusive. Attempts to alleviate chronic glaucoma by means of sedatives and tranquillizers seem to us to have been notably unsuccessful, although in an occasional patient some benefit may have resulted.[1]

From this short and indecisive statement, we can see the workings of the traditional medical mind. First of all, the entire notion of emotional causation is brushed aside simply because 'the evidence looks quite inconclusive'. Secondly, the attempts to alter emotional habits with patients were limited to the grossest, and most unsuccessful, form of emotional treatment, that of sedative and tranquillizer treatment. Even in considering emotional causation, doctors still have nothing to offer but the ingestion of drugs for altering a condition of anxiety or stress.

What do we begin to see when we take a closer look at the nature of anxiety? First of all, the word itself comes from the old German *angst*,

[1] G. K. Krieglstein, *Glaucoma*, page 7 (New York, 1983).

which originally meant 'a choking in the narrows'. This term not only defines anxiety, it also exactly defines what happens in the trabecular meshwork!

If we consider for a moment that glaucoma is not an isolated incident in the eye, but a general expression of a condition of the whole person, what do we find? A person who is anxious is holding in emotions, rather than letting them flow out. Anxiety is a blocking of an outward movement of the feelings. It is a constriction. We see this constriction in the diaphragm muscle, the chest muscles, the throat particularly, the vocal chords and tongue – so why not assume it could develop in the visual centre as well?

In fact, it makes sense to assume that a condition of constriction and blocking seen almost everywhere else in the body would also manifest itself in the ocular region, because this is a primary location for the expression of emotions. If a person is afraid to express anger, for instance (the usual emotion behind the anxiety) the blocking must stop a vocal discharge through the mouth, a physical discharge through the arms and legs (hitting and kicking for instance), *and* the powerful expression of the anger through the look in the eyes.

We all know that our eyes can be expressive of emotion. Phrases like 'if looks could kill', 'she nailed him to the spot with her glare', 'the look in her eyes melted my heart', and so on, indicate that there is an observable expression of feelings that flows out through the eyes.

Take a young child with traditional parents who do not allow the overt expression of anger in the home. The child will naturally become angry when frustrated – this is an instinctual reaction. Punishment ensues. After a number of such incidents, the child becomes angry, but instantly fears punishment for the expression of the anger. Step by step, tensions block the free expression of the emotions, until the feelings no longer flow freely out from the body.

Usually, the last blocking to take place with a child is in the eyes. You have certainly witnessed the following scene: a 4-year-old has learned to block his of her anger vocally and physically. But still, the child stands there with pent-up anger, the body frozen rigid but the eyes glaring with heated emotions. And the mother or father then notices this visual expression, and punishes the child for the expression in the eyes. 'Don't you look at your mother like that!' is an almost universal phrase in families, at least in good Christian families where anger is not accepted in children.

The point is this – the child had to learn to stop the emotional flow to the eyes. Constriction was essential to avoid punishment. I propose that when the child successfully developed the habit of blocking the

---

[1] *Glaucoma*, page 7.

expression of emotions through the eyes that child at that point became a likely candidate for developing glaucoma later in life.

Such emotional/muscular constrictions usually take years before they finally result in a physical disease or complication. But we need to look to the heart of the situation, to see if there is a positive opening to understanding the cause of glaucoma. What do you think? Do the emotions affect the functioning and the health of the body? Is it possible that emotional constriction resulting in physical constriction could lead to the blocking and constriction of the trabecular meshwork?

At this point, all indications point in this direction. But we cannot approach such a causal factor from a purely medical angle. Doctors have two paths at their disposal – surgery and drugs. These are the great gifts they have to contribute to our health and well-being – extreme measures when the system has already broken down. But when it comes to approaching the emotional make-up of a human being, medical science is almost totally ill-prepared to assume such a responsibility. For this reason, perhaps, it has taken us so long to arrive at seemingly simple insights into the causal mechanisms of disease. You need a supporting philosophy in order to function practically. And the medical philosophy, as sound and practical and helpful as it is in treating extreme conditions of disease, simply does not offer a foundation upon which to make this next step.

It should be once again pointed out that certainly, particular doctors and professors in the medical world are now making this step from 'Newtonian' medicine to 'Einsteinian' medicine. The primary problem with medical education and training is that it requires so much memorization and conceptual work, there is simply no time, space, or energy left for the doctor to develop an expanded understanding of health based on the holistic notion of human organisms. We are seeing the breakdown of the traditional medical system, as you are most likely aware. But at the same time, evolution carries on, and new forms rise up, often right in the middle of the medical community.

I say these last words so that it is obvious that I am not attacking the medical profession. If they had a functioning model explaining reasonably the causes of glaucoma, there would be no difficulty. But the problem is that there exists no working medical model which helps us treat glaucoma more successfully than drug administration and symptom treatment. So we have no choice but to take a step back, try to see a larger view of the situation, and integrate several equally significant models into one working structure. I feel we are close to this integration with such an emotional-causation theory of glaucoma.

The obvious question, however, is how does such a theory develop into a practical programme which glaucoma patients can apply successfully to their particular condition? How can the blocking pattern be reversed, the emotional inhibitions loosened, and the habitual constrictions eased?

As with the other alternative programmes presented in this book, a common theme prevails: consciousness seems to be an essential, powerful factor in the recovery from disease. Our attitudes influence the way our bodies function. So we can work directly with our consciousness to alter a glaucoma condition for the better.

But please notice the vast difference in this approach to the medical approach: in traditional medicine, the patient is the passive victim, putting all his trust and hope in the actions of the external agent, the doctor and the doctor's drugs. Healing is a process instigated by the intervention of the doctor/priest, with the helpless patient looking to the will and consciousness of the doctor to bring it about.

Does healing actually take place in this manner?

If disease is caused by external agents, with the ill person an innocent victim of chance infection, etc., then an external agent could enter the picture and do battle with the external agent causing the disease.

But if disease is caused by unconscious emotional constrictions and negative thought patterns generated by the consciousness of the patient him or herself, then it must be the patient who acts directly, to heal him or herself.

I am not stating this as gospel truth, I am simply putting the idea out for you to consider for yourself, from your unique point of view. Does this logic ring true for you? Do you have the ability actively to heal yourself?

Our belief systems limit us totally. Basically, we can function only within the limitations of what we believe to be true. If we don't think we can heal ourselves, if we feel that we are helpless victims, then certainly, we will have no luck in consciously acting to reverse negative patterns in the body. Only as our beliefs expand as our culture grows, can we change the health situation we are confronted with.

With this book and its glaucoma programme, you can gain an understanding of an alternative concept for mind/body integration. Quite possibly you are already developing this expanded belief in your own personal potential, and this book is simply pointing to particular illnesses where you can apply your evolving confidence in your healing potential.

In any case, the following programme provides the basic structure for a glaucoma recovery programme, focused primarily on the most common form of glaucoma, primary open-angle glaucoma. But the basic principles will readily transfer to the other glaucomas as well.

If you want an expanded programme on cassette tape, you can

obtain two half-hour programmes which have been designed to powerfully guide you through the learning process of focusing your mind's full attention directly to the spot in the body which really needs your attention, love, and healing energy.

THE GLAUCOMA RECOVERY PROGRAMME

You will want to review Chapter 5 as a beginning to this programme, and especially to explore the exercises of Personal Power, Fear/Assertion, the Inner Smile, and Facing Your Danger. Chapter 6 also contains key exercises. Glaucoma definitely seems to be associated with tension, anxiety, and chronic breath inhibitions. Be sure to consider this dimension of healing, before advancing to the following healing session.

You have glaucoma. Constriction blocks the flow of liquid through the trabecular meshwork. The physical alteration required for you to reduce your eye pressure is as follows: the tension and constriction of the trabecular meshwork, or related conditions explained by your doctor, must relax, expand, by more porous and vulnerable, and allow the emotional excitation to flow through the eyes once again. To encourage this development, you can regularly devote yourself to the following experience.

Find a quiet place where you can rest undisturbed for twenty minutes to half an hour. Be sure you are relaxed, comfortable, warm, and free of immediate obligations.

Sit or lie down, whichever you prefer for this session, and bring your focus to your breathing.

Simply be aware of the air as it goes in and out of your nose. Feel the actual physical sensation, and allow that sensation to bring you deeply into contact with your inner workings.

Relax your feet, tense them and then let them relax even deeper. Do this with your right leg now. And now your left leg. Tense it. Then relax it, exhaling deeply, with a sighing sound.

Now allow this relaxation to move up your body, into your pelvis. Tense your sexual region, and then let it relax. Feel the soft flow of relaxation and warmth flooding up your body, with every breath increasing and feeling more enjoyable.

Allow this feeling of relaxation to move up into your chest, as your diaphragm muscle relaxes on a deep exhalation, and your chest sighs with the peace and calmness.

Feel your heart in your chest. Allow it to relax. Hold your focus on your heart and simply watch what feelings might arise.

Allow this awareness to move up towards your throat now. Breathe through the mouth so that you open your throat more. Make any sounds that might want to come out, sighing and yawning perhaps.

Let your jaw relax, and your lips. Feel your tongue relaxing inside your mouth. Breathe into this sense of growing relaxation and also notice the increased flow of energy and vitality you might feel moving up through your body.

Now allow your awareness to move into your head, into the actual space where your brain is. Breathe into this focus, experience directly the presence of your brain, the centre of your consciousness.

And gently, effortlessly, allow your awareness to expand out into your eyes themselves. Breathe so that your whole body brings its focus to your eyes.

Be aware of them in your head, notice any tensions, and allow that tension to relax. You might want to tense your eyes tightly closed a moment, and then sigh as you relax them.

Play with the feeling of breathing in and out through your eyes as well as your nose or mouth. With every inhale, feel that you are taking in healing energy from the outside. And with every exhale, send your healing energy out to your eyes.

Feel the slight movement of your eyes as you breathe in, and then breathe out. Be relaxed and gentle with yourself, not pushing anything, just watching, focusing, encouraging.

Now bring your focus to the area just behind your cornea, to the aqueous humour and the ciliary body. Hold your attention there without effort. Don't try to make anything happen, just observe what happens.

Feel the presence of the aqueous humour as it is secreted from the ciliary body into the aqueous chamber. Be conscious of this process. Be open to any feelings that you might have, and allow yourself freedom and permission to express them.

And bring your awareness to the pressure inside your eyeball. Just look, experience, focus. Accept yourself as you are right now. Trust that you can heal naturally.

And now allow yourself to feel the aqueous humour flowing down through the trabecular meshwork, filtering gently through the porous tissues as they open up, relax, and let go of their habit of being tight and constricted.

To whatever extent you are ready to today, surrender to the new opening which is coming to you, to the relaxation and natural flow of the aqueous humour down out of the eyes, and the natural flow of your emotions out through your eyes.

Stay with this new feeling, explore the unique sensations, say hello to old feelings which you blocked, and simply let yourself relax further into this peaceful state of recovery, of acceptance, of evolution.

Let the tears flow if you want to, and express any feelings of anger with your voice, your arms and legs, and especially with your eyes. Don't force anything, simply surrender to your natural healing process, both emotionally and physically.

And when you are ready, you can end this session whenever you want, and return to normal consciousness as you go about your day.

15 • CROSS-EYES AND WANDERING EYES (Strabismus)

One of the remarkable features of the human visual system is its ability to direct both eyes at a single point in space, so that a true stereoscopic image is received in the brain.

The experience of three-dimensional space is created through looking at an object from two different points of view, at the same time. The distance between our two eyes creates this stereoscopic perspective.

The muscles which control the movement of each eye are called the extraocular muscles, as discussed in Chapter 1. When we want to look at a particular point in space, the muscles of both eyes receive identical orders from the brain, so that both eyes turn equally together. This linked muscular coordination of the two eyes is what makes stereoscopic vision possible.

But unfortunately for a small percentage of us, this linking mechanism does not function properly. The eyes do not work in harmony to point together at the same point in space, and so stereoscopic vision does not exist.

Instead, one eye (the dominant one) is directed at the desired object in the environment, while the other eye is looking elsewhere. The other eye is usually crossed, or looks off to one side, as shown in the illustrations. This general condition is called strabismus, or alternatively, amblyopia.

We have all seen people with this condition, and it is often a complicating factor in relating. Sometimes we don't know which eye the person is looking through, so we don't know if he or she is looking at us directly, of perhaps looking off somewhere else, where the other eye is aimed. The embarrassment works both ways, of course. People with wandering eyes often have difficulty in relating, because of this complication.

There are many complex varieties of strabismus, and much confusion still exists as to the cause of the condition, and the proper treatment. Children are often born with cross-eyes or wandering eyes, and treatment schedules are difficult to determine.

Before the advent of modern surgical medicine, very little could be

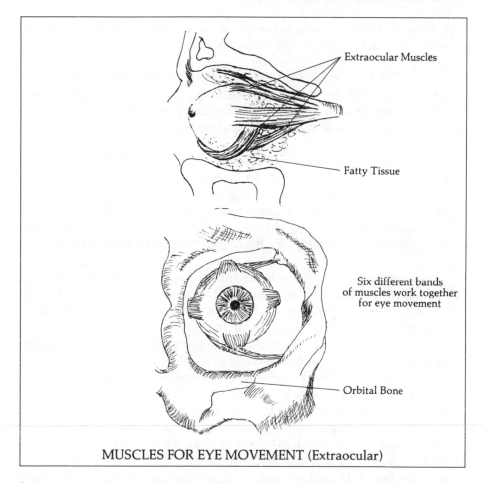

Extraocular Muscles

Fatty Tissue

Six different bands
of muscles work together
for eye movement

Orbital Bone

MUSCLES FOR EYE MOVEMENT (Extraocular)

done to correct strabismus. The person with the condition would naturally start favouring the use of one eye over the other, so that the brain would not be confused by two different images seen at the same time. So one eye would become dominant, and the other eye would fall into disuse.

Unfortunately, especially in childhood when the eyes are still developing, the eye which is not being consciously used can atrophy in the retinal and optic nerve regions, and become permanently blind. Then if there is damage to the dominant eye, vision is lost altogether.

This is one of the primary reasons that modern doctors encourage early operations on children with strabismus. Through surgery on the extraocular muscles, the eyes can often be brought into stereoscopic harmony, and full use of both eyes becomes possible. Through putting an eye patch over the dominant eye, the lazy, wandering, or crossed eye can be forced to work again, and after the surgical correction of the muscular balance, full vision is recovered.

However, there are many complications to this procedure, and we should take a step back and consider this condition in a little more depth.

One of the reasons that eyes cross should definitely not be approached through surgery, for example. We have already discussed hyperopia, or far-sightedness caused by an eyeball which is too short in length. When a person with this condition looks up close, the eyes very often cross.

This is caused by an over-reaction of what we call the converging mechanism of the eyes. When we look in the distance, both eyes are looking in parallel directions, as shown in the illustration on page 9. But when we look up-close, the eyes lose their parallel position, and both look inward towards the centre. The closer we look, the more convergence there must be for both eyes to fixate on the same spot in space.

A remarkable mechanism links this convergence behaviour of the eyes with the focusing, or accommodative, mechanism which must also shift in order to focus up-close. As the brain sends orders to the ciliary muscles to tense so that the lens in each eye will focus up-close, a linked set of orders go to the muscles surrounding the eyes, generating proper convergence for that particular focal length.

All works wonderfully, unless the shape of the eye is too short, causing the ciliary muscles to have to contract much more strongly than normal to bring the close object into focus. If the focusing apparatus is working twice as hard to focus, then the extraocular muscles will automatically work twice as hard in convergence. The result is cross-eyes when looking up-close.

The proper optometric treatment for this condition is corrective glasses which reduce the focusing power needed to see up-close. When the ciliary muscles no longer have to contract abnormally to focus up-close, the linked muscles surrounding the eyes no longer over-react to create cross-eyes, and all is well.

Some children, for reasons still unknown and perhaps linked to emotional growth, recover from hyperopia as they mature, and can then put away the glasses and also maintain straight eyes. For those who do not recover, contact lenses can be used to lessen the difficulty of wearing corrective lenses.

Another related condition sometimes develops, which is still a convergence problem, but not related to actual eye dysfunction at all. Instead, the brain itself fails to perform the convergence work correctly. Instead of a one-to-one ratio between focusing and convergence, the brain might employ a two-to-one ratio, for instance. The eyes would over-react to focusing up-close, and cross-eyes would result.

Traditionally, this condition has been considered a purely neurological complication, and bi-focals are prescribed to do the focusing all the time for the eyes. When there is no visual impulse to focus close-up, there is no over-reaction of the extraocular muscles, and cross-eyes do not occur.

At times, doctors prescribe special eye drops which help the eyes focus with less effort, through reducing the size of the pupil. It is not well-understood how this reduction lessens the work of the focusing mechanism, but sometimes the eye drops succeed in stopping the cross-eye reaction.

The other most common cause of both cross-eyes and wandering eyes is a muscular defect. As we have seen earlier, each eye has six muscles which control the direction and movement of the eye. These muscles are connected to a point behind the eyes, and work in opposite pairs to generate movement of the eyes.

To look in one direction, for instance, one of the muscles of a pair relaxes, while the other tenses an equal amount. Movement is thus generated. A complex co-ordination of all six muscles generates accurate aiming of the eye in the desired direction.

But if a child is born with, or develops, muscles which are of unequal length and/or strength, the tug-of-war between the paired muscles will result in an imbalance, and the eyes will not naturally function correctly for stereoscopic vision. This condition is not usually correctible with glasses, and is dealt with through eye exercises and/or surgery.

For many years now, surgeons have been operating on the extraocular eye muscles, in order to correct, or at least reduce, the muscle imbalance which generates the cross-eye and wandering eye condition. These operations continue to become more complex and successful, although there are many cases where incorrect surgery permanently damages the muscular potential of the patient.

What does the operation actually entail? In simple form, the surgeon wants either to shorten the muscle slightly, so that it will pull the eye more in its direction, or to lengthen the opposite muscle, so that it does not exert quite so strong a pull. As a general rule, surgeons prefer to strengthen a weak or short muscle by moving its location on the surface of the eyeball, rather than weakening the opposite muscle. At times, both muscles are operated on.

Also, there are many operations where both eyes are operated on, in equal manner, so that the eyes both alter their muscular function in the direction of stereoscopic vision.

These operations require both surgical precision, and also an intuitive touch, because there is no specific guideline for how much alteration in muscle position generates a particular alteration in eye movement. Each person is unique, and the surgeon must guess exactly what surgical procedure is going to result in the desired effect. The normal ratio predicts that for every millimetre that a muscle is set back five degrees of correction will result. But the size and tonus of the muscle will determine variations in this rule of thumb, and the surgeon, when operating, must inspect the muscles and make a rapid guess at the exact operation to be performed.

Because of this uncertainty, the operation often results in over-correction, or under-correction, and yet another operation must be made to fine-tune the condition towards stereoscopic vision.

The operation itself takes from half an hour to an hour and a half. Children usually receive full anaesthetic and are asleep during the operation. Adults usually can be operated on with only local anaesthetic and a tranquillizer. In general, you can go home the same day as the operation, suffering only from the temporary pain of the incision into the eye, which is taken care of by pain-killers, and the lingering effects of the anaesthetic.

It is accepted practice to operate on a child at the early age of six months, and considerable controversy remains as to the proper age for operating, because sometimes, spontaneous correction of the condition occurs. You are well-advised to consult at least two physicians before determining if and when to have your own child operated on.

For many years, the alternative to surgical intervention has been visual therapy, where eye exercises are performed over and over again, in an attempt to teach the muscles of the eyes to perform their function correctly. Especially in the United States, visual therapists are much in evidence.

If you ask a surgeon about visual therapy for treating cross-eyes and wandering eyes, he will usually laugh and tell you not to waste your time. His argument is that children especially simply won't dedicate themselves to the exercises, and even if they did, the results indicate that visual therapy is usually ineffective.

Visual therapists, of course, will tell you a totally different story. They are, for the most part, very dedicated human beings, working patiently hour after hour with both children and adults, helping them to perform visual movements which lead in the direction of better visual functioning.

The difficulty with visual therapy is that it treats only 50 per cent of the problem. As we have seen throughout this book, our eyes and our emotions are intimately linked. Visual therapy treats the muscular, physical condition present, but almost never is there treatment for the emotional condition which either generated the condition in the first place, or developed as a result of the genetic defect.

Thus, a person with a wandering eye consciously wants to work to bring that eye into correct alignment, but perhaps unconsciously wants to maintain the condition. And children with visual co-ordination problems might be forced to do the exercises, but emotionally might maintain a reaction against seeing clearly with the 'bad eye'. Thus the will to see clearly battles with the emotions fearing this clarity, making visual therapy much less effective than it could be with proper emotional counselling and breath recovery therapy.

Once again, we find ourselves against the same medical wall. Eye doctors are not trained in emotional therapy, and they tend mostly to deny the causal factors of emotional stess and prolonged fear patterns in the development of any visual problem. For them, strabismus is almost entirely a genetic, inherited defect, and the proper correction is through surgery or optics. Certainly, there are enlightened doctors who are balancing hereditary with emotional and environmental factors, and are looking for signs of emotional causation.

But unfortunately, therapy techniques for reversing emotional contractions and habitual physical conditions are still in their infancy and are seldom available. So even if a doctor might suspect that a child's vision problem has been caused by emotional trauma, he sees no alternative but surgery for correction of the problem.

The difficulty naturally arises if surgery corrects a physical disorder, but the underlying emotional disorder remains. Will the body generate a substitute pattern to maintain the blocking created with stabismus? Very often, when working with people who have received the strabismus operation and now have supposedly stereoscopic vision, I find that in fact, they are still not using the old wandering eye, even though it now physically functions correctly. And even if they do see through the eye, very often there is no emotional linkage with that eye. The deeper blindness remains.

At a conference for visual therapists, I once went around asking experienced therapists what they could tell me about the breathing habits of children with cross-eyes. Except for one therapist, none of them had made a mental note of how their hundreds of patients breathed. The one who had noted breathing, a therapist also trained in psychology, instantly stated what I have found to be the universal case also – people with strabismus demonstrate an inhibited breathing profile. They breathe almost exclusively in the chest, tend to hold their breath at the top of their inhalation, and have very weak and partial exhalation. The breathing is irregular, movement of the pelvis during respiration is almost totally blocked, and the movement of air through the throat is audible, indicating chronic tension of the vocal cords.

The muscles of the breathing apparatus are primary muscles of the body, instinctively maintaining optimum levels of oxygen in the bloodstream. Fear, tensions, stress, anxiety and rejection generate an inhibition of the spontaneous breath response.

Curiously, fear is also linked with a particular contraction of the eye muscles. If someone is suddenly frightened intensely, the eyes instinctively roll up in the head, and the convergence mechanism is activated in the extreme, creating a temporary case of radical cross-eyes. The breathing freezes on the inhale, and the diaphragm muscle which must relax for a full exhalation of power, is caught in chronic tension.

Is there a relationship between cross-eyes, and early-childhood trauma which generated chronic states of apprehension in the baby? Is there a direct linkage between the instinctual reaction of fear in the eyes and the habit of cross-eyes?

Parents never want to consider that they may have done something that would injure their child. This is one of the great fears of parents, and doctors are very careful not to raise the question of parent responsibility. This is quite unfortunate, because it blocks the logical thinking processes which would explore both the emotional causes of physical disorders, and also their reversal.

It is well-documented that the emotional condition of a mother while carrying her baby in the womb influences the development of the foetus. Both diet and emotional condition affect the uterine condition. A baby in the womb is certainly affected by a mother who is in constant anxiety. This anxiety is picked up by the nervous system of the child, surely, and is translated into the physical manifestation of the fear.

So a child who is born cross-eyed – is this purely a genetic, inherited condition, or was pre-natal anxiety a factor in the visual abnormality? The answer to this question has not been researched adequately as yet, but the indications point towards a strong relationship between womb conditions and the development of post-natal complications.

We assume that children are helpless victims of their genetic inheritance. When we see a poor little girl with her eyes hopelessly crossed, we feel compassion for her, sorry for her.

But perhaps we are doing her a serious disservice with all this pity. Perhaps we would shift her entire condition if we began to consider if she were responsible for the condition herself. As long as she is seen as a victim, and is taught to see herself in this way, she will never consider the possibility that she is somehow generating the condition, and that therefore she has some power to reverse it.

Unless we assume responsibility for creating our physical states, we cannot assume responsibility for reversing that condition. I am not talking about guilt, however. Guilt is a judgement against ourselves. Assuming responsibility is simply accepting the reality of the situation, and regaining our sense of power to alter the situation.

Almost never have I heard of a doctor, therapist, or parent who asked a cross-eyed child why they were looking the way they were, or who asked them why they didn't want to see with both eyes. Also, almost never have I heard of a doctor or therapist who patched the dominant eye and then related to the child through the other eye, to make direct contact with the part of the child that was basically looking away from reality. These are simple therapy techniques, but they can produce sudden, dramatic results.

What usually happens is that a child is forced to wear a patch over the dominant eye, before the strabismus operation, so that the weak eye will be forced to work. But no emotional exploration or support is offered to the child at this point. The poor child has suddenly to face the blocked feelings related with this eye alone, and further emotional trauma and blocking will often result.

Our problem is that we are all afraid of our hidden monsters and bogey-men. We grew up and pushed away our childhood fears, buried them deep and ran away from them. And the last thing we want is to be brought back in contact with those fears through accepting the fears of a child. To be open to letting a child express her or his fears, requires that we are open to our own. And for most of us, this is simply not the situation.

So children are left alone with their fears. They must somehow deal with them, overcome them, or block them. Such conditions as strabismus, myopia, eye allergies, and the like very probably are a result of this factor of childhood fears.

For a parent of a cross-eyed or wandering-eyed child, the first step is not to seek help for the child, but to look to yourself. Certainly, take the child to the doctor and proceed as seems most reasonable with the visual condition. But also look to see if your own fears have perhaps rubbed off in your child.

We speak of genetic inheritance of family traits. But we also inherit the emotional traits of our family, generation after generation. From the womb, we pick up basic contractions, and also basic expansions, and are born with these predispositions. Only through consciously looking at ourselves, can we see our emotional inheritance, and begin to move beyond contractions which do not benefit us.

And breath patterns are the crucial indicators. Our breathing automatically reflects our emotional condition, unless we learn to block this. If your child has cross-eyes and also seems to breath shallowly, in the chest, unevenly, and with tensions, you know that help is needed not just for the eyes, but for the breathing as well. Some useful books are listed in the bibliography.

To finish this regrettably short discussion of strabismus, I would recommend that you take a step back from your accepted notions of the condition, and simply look at the problem from the point of view that includes emotional factors as well as genetic. Be open to the possibility that a person with the condition might be able to recover if allowed to release the emotional tensions that sometimes stand behind the condition. And look to your own emotions to see if they are reflected in the child.

If you are grown up, or even a child but ready to look into yourself honestly, you should begin to approach your wandering eye, or your 'bad eye', in a new light. Cover your dominant eye regularly, and while remaining aware of your breathing, explore what feelings are associated with the bad eye.

In this chapter as throughout this book, I do not mean to in any way disregard the great contribution which medical science has made to the treatment of visual disorders. My intention is not to criticize surgical and medication treatments, but to suggest where further advances might be possible.

Certainly, genetic inheritance is a factor in all of our lives. Children are definitely born with defects which are not just of emotional origin. My suggestion is that we would be more effective in our treatments if we considered the interaction of genetic and emotional factors in any disease, and developed techniques which integrated medical and psychological approaches.

Perhaps most importantly, I am suggesting that we treat the eyes as being intimately related to the rest of the mind/body continuum, instead of approaching them as isolated organs untouched by such factors as breath inhibitions, emotional phobias, and thought patterns.

And finally, when we treat a person as a victim, we make that person a victim. When we give a person responsibility for his or her own body, we give that person the power to become more healthy. Only with this sense of personal integrity can self-healing take place. If the emotional factors are considered and recovery does not follow, then certainly, surgery is invaluable. But we must at least reflect upon and actively explore the alternatives.

16 • EYE ALLERGIES
(Conjunctivitis)

The outside surface of the eye is covered with a thin membrane called the conjunctiva. This protects the cornea from damage and also takes in oxygen for the cells of the cornea to utilize..

Eye allergies are usually caused by a reaction of the cells of the conjunctiva to a foreign substance which lands on the conjunctiva surface is called an allergen, because of its ability to generate an allergic reaction.

Specifically, the allergen comes into direct contact with a chemical called IgE which is bound to certain cells in the conjunctiva, and this contact generates the release of protective chemicals called histamines, and related substances.

The histamines actually cause the condition we know of as an eye allergy. They have an effect on local blood vessels, causing dilation and redness, and on secretory glands as well. This process is extremely complex, and if you want the biochemical explanation, you can read such books as *Allergy and Immunology of the Eye*[1] for the full story.

For our purposes in this book, we want to explore why certain people react with this allergic response to allergens, while most people do not. Furthermore, we will want to see what traditional medical treatments are most effective against this reaction, and what alternative treatments can be employed with success.

The most common eye allergy is associated with a more general bodily reaction called hay fever. Many foreign substances can cause this reaction of sneezing, itching, runny eyes and nasal obstruction. Pollens such as ragweed, timothy grass and other grasses, and pollen from such trees as elm, poplar, oak, birch, cedar, and juniper have been identified as allergens.

Moulds can also be allergens which generate hay fever. And indoor irritants such as dust mites, cat, dog, horse, rabbit, and mouse hair, can be allergens, as well as feathers and wool. Insects can also generate an allergic response, such as the caddis fly.

Organic dusts from green coffee, wood, tannic acid, cotton seed,

[1]D. D. Natan (Boston, 1982).

flours, and grains can lead to conjunctivitis, and industrial chemicals such as platinum salts, nickel salts, and penicillin are known allergens for some people.

Some of these, especially the pollens, are seasonal, and cause attacks only for a month or two each year. Others are present all year round.

For simple hay fever attacks, antihistamines are usually prescribed by doctors. These inhibit that initial reaction we discussed earlier in the chapter, and thus block the resultant inflammation, itching, burning, and mucous discharge. These antihistamines must be used regularly to be effective, and have a secondary, complicating sedative effect. Caffeine and other stimulants are usually included to balance this sedative effect.

An alternative treatment to drugs for hay fever is the therapy called hypo-sensitization. This technique requires the identification of the offending allergen, and the repeated injection of small quantities of this allergen into the body. The result is often the development of an immunity to the substance.

Ragweed allergy is especially responsive to this form of treatment, as are other grass pollens and sometimes house dust. But the treatment is often ineffective, or the body then develops other allergies to replace the original one. We see with allergies, as with other conditions, the dimension of emotional causation present. This will be discussed in a moment.

Another variation on the hay fever theme, directly related to pollens and other allergens, is called atopic conjunctivitis. The condition can be extremely painful, especially with itchiness and scratchiness. Attacks are sudden and often visually disabling. Medication with antihistamines is sometimes effective, and using corticosteroids is effective but with complications in long-term use. Vasoconstrictors are also helpful.

This condition is usually developed during childhood, and curiously often goes away with maturity, indicating some linkage with emotional trauma during puberty. It is a hypersensitivity syndrome, an over-reaction to an irritant.

A very similar condition, vernal conjunctivitis, shows the same symptoms, but seems to be generated simply by warm weather, appearing in the spring, in warm climates especially.

This condition affects boys twice as often as girls, a statistic unexplained by medical knowledge. It can be almost unbearably painful, as sharp growths on the conjunctiva regularly scratch the inner eyelid with every movement of the eye and every blink. The attacks last perhaps an hour, and then often disappear for hours or days.

There are numerous drugs now on the market for treating this condition and related allergic reactions.

The contraceptive drugs which are taken regularly to build up a blocking mechanism to allergens are most popular, some of which are available without prescription. Consultation with a doctor is recommended if the condition is serious, since some of the over-the-counter treatments are less than ideal, and medical examination might show unusual conditions in the eyes that need to be treated.

However, apart from the application of drugs, medical science is still uncertain as to how to eliminate hypersensitivity. The traditional approach sees allergic reactions as a purely physiological condition, generated by hereditary weaknessess and biochemical malfunctions. The science of immunology has grown immensely, and is vastly complex and fascinating. But still, is this condition a purely biological disorder, or are there emotional components to it?

From the early days of psychotherapy, reports have linked hypersensitivities with emotional patterns. We can explore the basic understanding of allergies in this regard, and then see what practical steps can be made to deal with the psychological causes of allergies.

One case-study will give a general picture of the emotional-causation model to allergic reactions. A child with no previous allergic history suddenly developed extreme vernal conjunctivitis one spring. His eyes would become extremely scratchy, irritated, red, and painful, with great discharges of tears and stringy mucus. The burning would be almost impossible to stand, and total loss of normal functioning was effected until the attack receded.

This condition continued until the child grew up and left home and moved to another climate, when the attacks each springtime resided and then were gone. Only when he returned to his hometown area did the symptoms recur, except for unexpected periodic attacks which would last a week or so, and then be gone, with no relationship to geographic location or season.

In general therapy with me, this client gradually regained memory of this blank period of his past, and the real story emerged. At the time the child developed the allergy, his uncle was dying of a horrible disease, the physical effects of which were very disturbing to look at. Every afternoon that first spring when the allergy developed, the boy had to return home and visit the uncle.

The attacks stopped these visits. As he found it time to leave school and go home, his eyes would create such a trauma that the visit was regularly avoided. The lingering disease went on for years – as did the conjunctivitis.

Along with this avoidance pattern, the child remembered that he was not able to cry and show his grief over the beloved uncle's condition, because he had to be strong and support his mother, who was emotionally shattered by the disease of her brother. So the boy blocked the tears. Only when he had his allergy attacks did his eyes run with tears. But he had an excuse, the pain of the allergy attack.

In addition, he remembered how he felt his uncle's extreme pain in his own body, unable to block the feeling. His eye pain gave him an outlet through which to feel all this pain that was present in the household.

Finally the man remembered how he had felt left alone because his uncle got most of his mother's attention and sympathy. The development of the eye disease was a means of regaining some attention and care from the mother. If the eyes hurt badly enough, sympathy was switched from the uncle to the boy.

And so we see how a psychologist would evaluate the development of a hypersensitivity syndrome. He would respect the bio-medical model of the immunologists. But at the same time, he would place primary causative responsibility on the emotional situation of the child, not the genetic weaknesses or cellular malfunctions.

In more general terms, we can explore the following associations often made by therapists. First of all, when we consider the sneeze reflex which is activated by hay fever, we find that this powerful discharge is often a substitute for blocked emotions. The swelling of the nasal passageway is intimately linked with genital swelling during sexual arousal. Since boys develop hay fever twice as often as girls, is the fear of sexual arousal linked with sneeze attacks? Therapy cases indicate that this is so, at least in most cases.

And what about the blocking of the cry response in boys? Big boys don't cry, so the saying goes. The tears are held back. But then for some boys, a substitute is developed. With a hay fever attack, tears run freely. One shows almost identical symptoms of emotional release. But because hay fever is not culturally linked with emotional release, this is a safe way to discharge built-up emotions. Consciously, the child can feel a victim, and can surrender to the overwhelming attack of the allergy. But what is actually behind the attack?

Allergies are in fact attacks. Your conscious will is overwhelmed by the reaction to the environment, and there is no way to stop the discharge. You can be in a formal meeting with very respected dignitaries, but if you have to sneeze, you have to, even if the act is a great explosion that would appear to be a very violent gesture to the outside world.

And this shows another dimension of hay fever. It is a powerful, violent expression, perhaps releasing blocked angers at the outside world.

Whatever the analysis, we can see that hay fever would serve to allow emotions to be expressed safely, without being punished for their direct meaning, because both the victim of attack and the observers consider hay fever to be unrelated to emotional release.

What do you think?

And what can be done, aside from drug treatments, to reverse the hypersensitivity?

Basic emotional release therapy can be quite helpful for many allergy sufferers. When given the freedom to express buried emotions directly, quite often the substitute symptoms of allergic sensitivity disappear. This is facilitated by a trained therapist, especially in the Bio-Energetic tradition, but a friend can do much to help you also, and you can do much to help an allergic friend.

Simply sit and talk. Let the person remember his past, when he developed the allergy. See what comes to the surface. And especially, give her or him permission to release any emotions that might come up. Our fear of friends crying or releasing anger is one of the great problems in our society. Secondary medical problems so often develop because the primary emotional pressure was not allowed expression.

You can also do your own therapy. You can lie down for half an hour two or three times a week, alone, and breathe into whatever feelings might be rising to the surface.

ALLERGY RECOVERY SESSION

Specifically for an eye allergy condition, you can do the following session, which step by step helps you to break free of the habitual pattern of reacting to allergens. Even if you have worked through childhood emotions which established a pattern of hypersensitivity, the habit of over-reacting will remain until extinguished. This following session is a brief version of a deconditioning programme, using your direct mental intervention as the active ingredient.

Find a quiet place to sit or lie down, where you can be alone and undisturbed for twenty minutes to half an hour. Be sure you are comfortable and warm. If you have a tendency to fall asleep, sitting up is preferred.

Focus on your breathing. Watch the air as it goes in and out your nose. Expand your awareness to your head, and then to your whole body. Breathe into a growing sense of relaxation, as you feel your breathing expanding, slowing down, relaxing.

Now bring your awareness to your chest, and allow your attention to focus on the feelings inside your body. Let your allergy reactions come gently to the surface of your mind, as you remain focused also on your breathing and feelings.

See what memories begin to rise to the surface as you open yourself to experiencing events and feelings related with your early allergy attacks. Just see what comes now.

Continue to breathe into whatever memories come, and allow your emotions to be free to express the feelings that build up inside you.

Allow your eyes to respond to these feelings and memories. See what your eyes really want to do, and allow them to express your feelings as well as your breathing and your voice.

Stay aware of what is happening in your body. Feel your breathing leading you deeper and deeper into the depths of your allergic condition. Allow insights to rise to the surface now.

What emotions were you blocking through your allergic attacks? What feelings come to the surface now, as you give the emotions permission to express themselves?

Stay with your breathing, and allow the healing process to happen. Don't make any effort. Simply breathe into whatever comes.

And now we are going to focus on your habit of reacting too extremely to the irritants that stimulate your allergic reactions.

You no longer need to have this over-reaction. There is no need to hide your basic emotions. You can now let go of the over-reaction.

When you encounter an irritant that used to stimulate an allergic reaction, you can now choose not to over-react. You can let go of this habit.

Continue breathing, allow these words to sink deeply into your mind, down to where your automatic reaction centre is. Feel your consciousness moving down into the area where you store this habit of over-reacting to an irritant.

Move right into this area until you find the place where you store this linking of a particular irritant with an over-reaction.

State clearly that you no longer want this reaction to take place. Do not do this as a dictator, but rather as a friend. You are bringing good news. The body no longer needs to go through the painful allergy reaction. Let your whole body, throughout your millions and millions of cells, rejoice at this good news.

Feel a sense of relaxation developing, which brings about the final release of the old habit. Let off of the habit, thank it for trying to help you in the past, but make it clear that those times are gone for ever. Feel the joy and sense of release at this news, throughout your body.

And now allow this direct information to radiate out to the cells in your eyes, in the conjunctiva of your cornea. Allow the cellular functioning to respond to the new situation, so that when an irritant lands on the conjunctiva, there is no longer that initial reaction which generates histamines.

Instead, the cells of the conjunctiva will now tolerate irritants, absorbing them or letting them be washed away, but not setting off the allergic reaction any more.

Now relax, observe your breathing, and feel the sense of harmony and unity in your body. Allow your entire being to feel conscious at once, so that every cell in your body feels alive, integrated with your well-being, participating in a great organism which is now full of love, acceptance, and freedom of expression.

Continue to allow this feeling of well-being to radiate throughout your body, touching every cell. Feel your conjunctiva cells especially happy, freed from the abnormal reaction pattern which had caused them so much pain in the past.

Breathe into your new sense of wholeness. Feel your emotions integrated into your breathing, so that with every breath, you spontaneously release whatever you feel, so that no pressures develop.

And now relax, let whatever insights that want to rise to the surface do so. And when you are ready, you can open your eyes, stretch and yawn, and go on about your day, knowing that you have grown, and that your allergy is beginning to disappear.

Be sure to be patient, to do this session regularly, until the habit of your allergy is completely released, and you are free!

17 · THE RETINA: MIRACLES AND TRAGEDIES

We have now explored almost every major aspect of our eyes. We have seen how the shape of the eye and the curvature of the cornea can affect vision. We have taken a close look at the inner crystalline lens and the muscles which alter its focusing shape. We have considered the purpose and problems of the aqueous humour as it is created by the ciliary body and flows down through the front chamber of the eye. And we have seen how the extraocular muscles which surround and move the eyes make possible stereoscopic vision, and at times interfere with this vision. Except for the back sections of the eye, we have made a full survey of function, problems, and cures.

But we have still ahead of us a most remarkable aspect of vision, the actual processing of the light which enters the eye into electro-chemical information to be sent to the brain. And for this final phase of our journey, we find ourselves face to face with a seemingly miraculous region of the eye called the retina.

The retina is a thin, photosensitive layer of the eye, covering the inner surface of the back regions and held in place by the jelly-like substance which fills the back chamber of the eye. This jelly-like substance is called the vitreous humour, and we should first take a look at this rather large section of the eye, to see its relationship with the retina itself.

The vitreous humour, unlike the aqueous humour in the frontal chamber, is not in circulation. Instead of being regularly (every four hours) replaced by new liquid, it is a permanent jelly, serving the main purpose of holding the eye to its proper shape, and holding the retina in place in the back curved regions of the eye.

The vitreous humour is 98 per cent water. The other 2 per cent consists of a sponge-like structure which actually maintains the shape of the back of the eyeball. This sponge-like superstructure is attached to the retina, and any shifting of the position of the aqueous humour can affect the retina itself.

So we find the retina held in place from the front by the aqueous humour. It is also somewhat tenuously attached to the layer of the eye which is directly behind it, called the choroid. The choroid in turn is

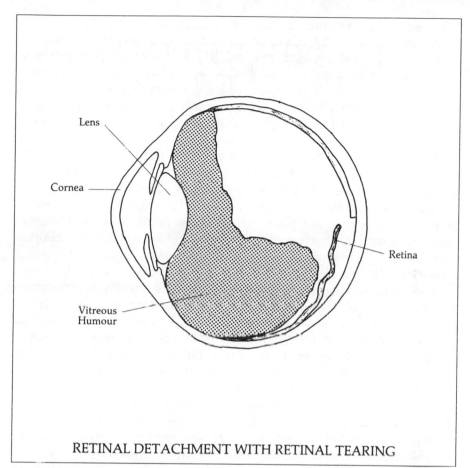

Lens

Cornea

Retina

Vitreous
Humour

RETINAL DETACHMENT WITH RETINAL TEARING

attached to the outer surface, or sclera, of the eyeball.

So if all goes well, the retina is firmly held in place, and maintains its constant position in the back of the eyeball. Let us look more closely now at the retina itself. I have been studying this part of the eye for a number of years already, and will certainly continue to study it for the rest of my life without fully understanding it, because our scientific grasp of its functioning is still in its infancy. The deeper we look, the deeper the mystery becomes. But this is true with all of science as we look at the infinite depths of the universe, and so for now we must be content with our present level of understanding.

The retina is only three cell-layers thick. This is extremely thin! The layer which rests against the choroid receives its blood supply and vital oxygen from the choroid blood capillaries. The outer layers, however, receive their blood supply directly from blood vessels serving this region of the retina directly. So in fact, there are two separate sources of blood for the retina, a fact which will become of critical note when we discuss various retinal complications.

The outer surface of the retina which is attached to the vitreous humour contains the photosensitive cells known as rods and cones, as mentioned in an earlier chapter. These two types of cells are capable of receiving the various light inputs which come from the outside world, and of translating this light energy into an electro-chemical signal which is sent to the brain for processing and for the final experience of seeing.

There is one very small part of the retina which is most sensitive to light signals. This is called the fovea, and it is here that we find a tight grouping of the colour-sensitive cells called the cones. If incoming light is focused on this small concentration of cells (about the size of a one-pence piece), then the optimum visual experience is possible. The outer cells are used for what we call periphery vision, when we notice the general full view coming into our eyes rather than focusing our attention to a specific spot.

You will remember our discussion in Chapter 2 when we mentioned the four modes of seeing – movement, form, colour, and space. When we look at the retina, we discover more precisely how this different seeing takes place. With movement, our brains are sensitive to all the inputs throughout the retina, looking to detect movement anywhere in the visual field. With perception of form, we are looking primarily with the fovea, seeing very clearly what we most want to see at a given moment, and then shifting to look with the fovea at a new spot. Colour seeing also uses the fovea primarily, but with an expanded field. And finally, when looking to see space, or to 'see everything at once', we are looking with an awareness of all inputs coming from the entire retina.

When it becomes dark, our cones can no longer detect the light stimuli we are receiving, and the rods, which are more in the periphery than in the fovea, come into play. Thus, our visual experience is quite altered when the sun goes down or we are in relative darkness. We will 'feel' differently, because our visual perception is in fact quite different. You might want to notice this consciously the next time you move from light to relative darkness.

Each cone or rod cell in the eye receives stimulation from the outside world, and then sends this information to the brain for processing. Actually, the first step of processing takes place in the retina itself, where groups of photo-receptors act together to determine relative shades of light and shadow, and then send this information along the optic nerve into the brain.

If the retina remains in place, receives a proper supply of blood, and maintains its communications link with the brain intact, clear vision is not affected at the retinal level.

But problems do arise with the retina, and we will consider the two main complications which many of us, especially as we approach old age, will fall victim to.

First of all, from a traditional medical viewpoint, old age itself is seen as a major cause of failing sight, related to retinal problems. The problem is actually not caused by the retina in this case, but by the vitreous humour we have just discussed. By the time we are 50 years old, it is estimated that 50 per cent of us will experience changes in the aqueous humour which can generate vision failure. By the age of 60 this figure has grown to two-thirds of the population. What is happening here?

The vitreous humour basically begins to collapse down inside the eye. The sponge-like structure releases some of its water, and drops down into the bottom of the eye, partly due to the life-time pull of gravity according to traditional theories. Actually, no one really knows what causes this collapse. But its effects can be quite drastic.

If the aqueous humour simply collapsed and fell away from the retina, there would be no major complications. But we have mentioned that the aqueous humour is connected to the retina, and as it collapses it can pull the retina away from the back of the eyeball. Actually, in most cases it is not the entire retina which pulls away from the choroid, but only a piece of it which breaks free from the rest of the retina and falls down with the vitreous humour.

The result is a hole in the retina. A number of holes can be created in this way, as the vitreous humour takes weeks or perhaps months to complete its collapse. These holes present the problem, because thay make an opening through which the water in the vitreous humour can seep in behind the retina, causing it to become detached from the choroid.

When this happens, the retina can fall forward from its proper position, and float aimlessly in the vitreous chamber. This obviously generates an impossible focusing situation in the eye, because the retina is not properly in line with the focusing mechanism anymore. The result is a loss of vision.

Another complication develops when the retina is separated from the choroid, because it then loses one of its primary sources of blood. This will obviously lead to a starvation of those retinal cells thus deprived of oxygen and nutrients. Unfortunately, the part of the retina which will die first will be the fovea, or macula, thus depriving the person of the ability to do detailed work. The peripheral vision can remain functional for over a year, but basically, the retina is in a very serious condition.

When this retinal detachment occurs, various symptoms are experienced. First one sees 'floaters' caused by debris and blood in the vitreous chamber. Then it seems that a veil has beeen pulled over one's eyes as the retina falls forward and down, eliminating any chance of clear focusing.

Obviously, when this happens the person with the retinal detachment experiences emotional trauma as the vision seems to fade away. Until the advent of modern surgical techniques, this loss of vision was permanent.

But recent innovations in eye surgery have generated considerable hope for recovery from this condition, and the sooner the surgical intervention, the more hope there is of returning the retina to its rightful place without too much cell damage. We can briefly explore the nature of this operation, so that you know the general procedure.

The first step in this surgery is to locate all of the holes which have developed in the retina. This in itself is a very difficult task, requiring high levels of magnification for detection.

The second step requires draining the water from behind the retina. A tiny hole is made through the outside of the sclera, and a tiny needle is pushed through the choroid itself, with infinite care not to rupture any blood vessels. Then when the needle is pulled out, the water can drain from this region and the retina will fall back into place.

The real trick of this operation is getting the retina to adhere to the choroid. The tissue is far too thin to use any needle and thread procedure, but another technique has been developed. The outside of the sclera is frozen or burned before removing the water behind the retina. When this frozen or burned region thaws out, it takes on a sticky, tacky quality from the irritation. And this serves to glue the retina back on to the choroid successfully. The outside of the eye is sometimes pushed forward against the retina to ensure adequate contact pressure, or the eye is bound with material to create a bulging towards the retina. This operation requires that the patient remain in bed for several days afterwards, and up to a week of quiet immobilization is usually recommended before the operation is considered complete and the person can go home.

This is quite a masterful operation reflecting the great advances in surgery which have been made over the last century. Nearly 90 per cent of these operations are successful with the first attempt, and a second or third operation usually serves for the majority of the remaining 10 per cent.

But retinal reattachment does not ensure clear vision. To the extent that retinal cells died during the detachment period, vision will of course be impaired. But the return of at least partial vision to the majority of patients with this condition is to be applauded.

As opposed to the more subtle, cellular dysfunctions we have encountered with such conditions as glaucoma and cataract, retinal detachment, once it occurs, does not appear to be in the realm of alternative healing. As with a broken arm or a lacerated leg, the definite physical injury needs definite medical intervention to correct the damage.

It is only when we begin to ask why the vitreous humour collapsed in the first place that we can begin to move in the direction of preventing this from happening. And what can be said has been said already in Part One: healthy diet, plenty of exercise, low-anxiety, and vital attitude all help to maintain optimum health of the visual system, including the vitreous humour.

DIABETES AND YOUR RETINA

We have now come, at the end of the book, to the most common cause of blindness in our culture today. We have also come to a discussion of the most rapidly spreading disease in our culture: diabetes. Specifically, diabetes mellitus.

There are 5–10 million diagnosed and undiagnosed diabetics in the United States alone, and this figure is doubling every fifteen years. Traditional theories as to this radical increase in the disease are linked to genetic factors. Because diabetic people are being kept alive so they can reproduce, so the theory goes, more and more diabetic genes are being transferred into the population, with the resultant increase in the disease.

This is certainly part of the picture. But we should at least briefly discuss the alternative point of view as to the cause of diabetes. This has to do with the stress factor in diabetes. In the same way that families pass on genes which can cause a weakness in the organs affected by diabetes, they can also pass on an emotional profile of chronic stress and over-arousal syndromes, which also seem to generate a failure in the organs associated with diabetes.

To what extent are diabetic genes proliferating in our culture, as opposed to the proliferation of stress and chronic arousal syndromes throughout the population? This is a question which needs to be determined, to really deal with the increase of diabetes in our communities and at large.

But such a discussion requires its own space elsewhere in the future. For our purposes here, we need to focus on the effects of diabetes on the visual system. Diabetes generates a predisposal to blindness which is twenty times that of the general population! The regular use of insulin serves to keep the diabetic alive and functioning normally, but the disease continues to cause physical problems, not only with the eyes, but with heart attack incidence, kidney problems, and poor circulation as well.

It is the circulation factor which most seriously affects a diabetic's eyes. There are two main developments which can occur, one which usually affects diabetics under 40, and the other which is usually found over this age. With the latter situation, the primary problem is that the capillaries which bring blood to the retina develop an unexplained tendency to leak blood, plasma, and fat-retaining materials, which then collect on the retina.

This leakage affects over 60 per cent of diabetics who develop retinal complications due to their disease, and is called background retinopathy. It does not generate total blindness, but causes a serious reduction in vision due to the covering of the retina with clumps of leakage.

The treatment for this condition requires the use of laser light. First, the surgeon must locate the leaks in the capillary system, and then he or she must spot-weld, or burn these holes closed.

The process is called photocoagulation, and can be done as an out-patient operation requiring only half an hour of actual surgery. Several operations might be needed to close all of the holes located in previous examinations. But once the holes are closed, the eye can begin to assimilate the leakage in the vitreous humour and on the surface of the retina, and clear vision can seemingly miraculously be regained. Periodic check-ups can catch any new leakage sites, which can be treated with photocoagulation as well.

The second primary problem with diabetes and the eyes, as mentioned before, affects younger people. There is no known explanation for this development, but for some reason, the capillary system in the retina begins to grow expanded networks in many younger diabetics' eyes, like a weed growing out of control. This condition, called proliferative retinopathy, leads to new blood vessels both in the retina itself, and also extending into the vitreous chamber.

Because these vessels are usually not very strong, they have a dangerous tendency to rupture, sending large amounts of blood into the vitreous humour. This blocks light from reaching the retina, and generates at least a temporary state of blindness in the affected eye.

Luckily, the eye will work to assimilate this blood, and after a period of time, the blood is cleared. But repeated ruptures will tax the removal ability of the eye, and at a certain point, blindness can develop permanently.

A curious and thus far mysteriously successful surgical treatment is now used for this condition. Rather than using individual laser beams to close individual leaks in the capillary system, as we saw earlier with background retinopathy, the treatment for proliferative retinopathy is far more radical. It is called panretinal photocoagulation and it involves firing 500—1000 beams at the retina in general, several different times, so that a total of 1500—3000 burns are generated at random spots throughout the retinal surface. The one area which is avoided is the optic nerve itself as it leaves the retina.

Overall, a full third of the retina is burned in this operation. This might seem drastic. But the operation is performed in the face of probable blindness due to the proliferation of the blood capillaries, and strangely enough, when one-third of the retinal surface is thus zapped, the brain sends messages to the capillary system to withdraw the newly developed capillaries, and the problem begins to recede, even around the optic nerve where there was no tissue damage.

Thus the condition, for a third of such patients, is reduced noticeably. For the second third the condition remains the same as before the operation, but no new growth develops. One-third, unfortunately, does not benefit from the operation. But it is considered worth the statistical risk to carry on with this operation, when permanent blindness is faced without such treatment.

There are, of course, many variations to the basic description I have given of the diabetic visual condition, and related operative techniques. The disease in general is under continual examination, and hopefully new breakthroughs will be made in the near future, further reducing the complications of the disease.

But we should finish this chapter with a positive look at what you can do for yourself if you are suffering from diabetes. It is a difficult condition, because you have been told of all the possible complications it could lead to. You can't help but worry about the possibility of visual complications suddenly striking you, forcing complex, expensive operations and perhaps leading to blindness in any event.

But if we step back and take a look at your condition from a broader perspective than statistical prediction and surgical intervention, what do we see?

We see your body suffering from the malfunction of one of your organs. You have been told that you are a helpless victim, and that you must simply accept your fate, take your daily medicine, and hope for as few complications as possible, as late in your life as possible.

You are certainly lucky to be living during a period when modern science can help you stay alive even though you have a traditionally deadly disease. But what can you do for yourself?

ALTERNATIVE APPROACHES TO DIABETES TREATMENT

There is obviously not room in a book such as this, for a complete discussion of the relationship between inherited stress and chronic arousal patterns, and the development of diabetes. This discussion and treatment programme is being prepared for another publication. What we can focus upon in this present chapter is a simple diabetic vision programme which you can use to explore your ability to heal yourself to whatever extent is possible.

Regardless of which specific visual dysfunction you might be suffering from, or if you have not developed a difficulty but know you might develop one, you can do a basic mind and body healing session to focus the proper state of consciousness on your eyes. We have been discussing this general approach throughout the book, so I will not repeat the premises behind the actual session.

Depending on your age, you know what retinal difficulties might develop, or have developed, in your particular case. Your challenge is to direct your mind to send orders, or requests, to the cells and tissue of your retina and vitreous humour, so that these complications do not develop, or are reversed if they have already begun. Thus you can put into specific words the more general guidelines offered in the following healing session.

Find a comfortable place to sit or lie down, where you will be undisturbed for twenty minutes or half an hour. Make sure you are warm, comfortable and free of distractions. Close your eyes, and begin to bring a focus to your breathing.

Watch how you are breathing now. Without judging or changing your breathing pattern, observe it and gain insight into your normal breathing habits.

Allow your breathing now to begin to relax step by step, as you let go of tensions and move into a more calm, open, centred state of mind and body.

After your next exhalation, make no effort to inhale at all. Simply hold your breath after the next exhalation, until the natural reflex to inhale grows inside you, deep down inside you, and you surrender to that inhale with effortless pleasure.

Do this several times. Explore that spontaneous impulse to inhale which comes when you simply exhale and watch what happens, making absolutely no effort to breathe at all.

Allow this effortless breathing to continue, as you remain aware of the centre deep within you which stimulates your next inhalation. Feel a growing sense of calm security coming into you, as you experience your inherent life-force which breathes you, even when you make no effort to breathe.

And now allow this feeling of natural vitality to move into the rest of your body, feel your organs relaxing, feel the stress slipping out of your body, as relaxation and vitality increase inside you with every inhalation of new life and peace.

And allow this peace and relaxation to rise up in your body, up through your chest and into your heart. Feel your heart beating in your chest, making no effort, simply putting your focus of attention to this powerful, lifelong pumping of blood throughout your body.

Maintain this focus on your heart, and simply observe your relationship with your heart. Allow whatever awareness is possible for you now, without forcing awareness at all. Accept yourself as you are, relax, and let the insights flow into your mind about your relationship with your heart.

Stay aware of your breathing, letting your exhalation be full, remaining empty until your spontaneous impulse to inhale brings the next breath of air into your lungs.

And now bring your awareness up through your neck. Relax your throat, your tongue, your vocal cords, and your jaw. Breathe through the mouth for a few breaths and feel your emotions free to come out if there is pressure inside you. Breathe into this pressure, and accept it, let it come out and be gone.

Now feel your awareness moving into your brain itself, filling that space inside your skull where your consciousness seems to be concentrated. Focus your attention directly to the centre of consciousness inside you. Do this effortlessly, with a sense of expansiveness, pleasure, and love for yourself.

And allow this awareness to move forward into your eyes now, gently, without effort, simply watching your breathing while at the same time allowing your awareness to expand to include your eyes.

Feel your eyes in their sockets. Move them around under your eyelids a little to be more aware of their presence. Hold your awareness on your eyes without force. See how you feel about this focus of attention. Accept whatever you discover about yourself, and remember there is plenty of time for growth and expansion.

Feel the blood your heart is pumping through your visual system now. Feel the flow, the movement, the regular pumping of blood to your retinas to keep the cells there alive and happy.

Stay aware of your breathing, notice what happens to your breathing as you focus on this basic bodily function. See how you feel about the nurturing of your eyes by your heart and breathing.

And now bring to mind the problems which might start to develop in your eyes, or which already are developing, and allow your consciousness to send suggestions to your eyes to reverse this development.

Breathe into this suggestion. Feel your consciousness flowing beautifully out to your eyes, out to the blood vessels which are in and around your retina. Allow the flow of orders and suggestions to reflect your general relaxation in your body.

Feel the health and vitality of your capillary system in your eyes expanding through this direct input of conscious energy and guidance, feel the love and compassion present.

And deep down in regions which are usually completely unconscious, allow yourself to feel a healing taking place inside you. Even if you have maintained your diabetic state from before you were born, allow yourself to feel a new sense of vitality coming into your body.

Breathe into this feeling, taking in health and relaxation with every inhalation, and blowing out stress and tensions with every complete exhalation.

See if you dare to heal yourself, to allow your whole body and mind to shift slightly towards health, integrity, vitality.

And relax, accept yourself as you are right now, and breathe into the possiblity that you can grow in directions which are not caught up in the diabetic tensions and failures. Feel whatever insights are rising to the surface now, be open to whatever feelings might need to break to the surface and be released. Surrender to the natural healing process which you have within you.

And when you are ready, you can open your eyes and stretch, and go on about your day!

18 · FINAL WORDS

Having followed light from its source in the heavens all the way through our visual system to its sudden explosion into consciousness, we can now relax, and perhaps reflect more spiritually and less medically.

Vision has not always been a medical specialization. For thousands of years on this planet, human beings have seen with eyes that looked beyond the mundane perceptions into what mystics see in dreams and children see in everything: the expanded perception where reality and vision intermix, and physical and spiritual dimensions find union.

So in our final words about vision, about how you see and how you can expand your perception in directions which bring more vitality and joy into your lives, we can mention vision as an aid to deeper seeing of the hidden meanings of life. We can let go of the diseases and distortions of our perceptual systems, and focus on the blessings and clarities which come to us through honest looking at the world around us.

When we see what we want to see, we don't really see at all. But when we risk really looking at what is in front of us, we encounter directly the vast infinity which is always there, waiting for us to open our eyes and see what life is really all about.

We are living on a planet which seems to be suffering from our very presence on its surface. We listen to the news and we read the papers and look around us at the problems which we face as a planetary civilization, and our vision seems struck with the danger and the fears and the overpopulation and all the rest.

But when we let go of our fears, when we completely exhale the old air, and allow our spontaneous life-force to bring a totally new inhalation of fresh air into our lungs, we find that we can see this reality in quite a different way. We can look around us and see what really needs doing, and instantly respond to fill the needs around us. Our eyes can learn to look in such ways that we act directly. And with this action, comes evolution, hope, and better times.

Joel Kramer, a man from whom I learned a great deal and who should be quoted with his clear and simple view of seeing, put it this way: 'It is not the desire to evolve that brings evolution, but rather the total seeing of oneself. Total seeing is what meditation is all about.'[1]

Total seeing has very little to do with the kind of clarity optometrists measure. A blind woman once told me that after she lost her eyesight, she finally found she could 'see' clearly. We have spent an entire book exploring ways in which you can see more clearly on the physical level. Certainly, this focus of attention is valuable, and I appreciate your reading through the book to understand the themes in their entirety.

But beyond one level there is always another dimension. This is the primary lesson of quantum physics as well as Tibetan Buddhism. No matter how deeply we look, the universe remains a remarkable mystery.

We have been looking at our ability to heal ourselves. We have been considering the possibility that human beings are evolving into a new period of history, where we break through our 'time barrier' of healing, or at least return to an earlier time when we understood it more deeply than we do at the present. I have attempted to integrate the new visions of medicine which are rising quickly into our culture with the traditional methods of medicine which are struggling ever more desperately to hold their own as the planet spins into a new era.

Now it is time for this book to come to an end, and for you to pause and reflect upon what insights might have come to your mind, through reading this book.

I am neither an eye surgeon nor a guru, and I do not pretend to have said the ultimate word either on medical approaches to vision problems nor on para-medical approaches. My aim has been to give you enough thought material so that you can carry on by yourself, exploring your healing potential while you deal with whatever conditions your eyes present to you.

The Sufi tradition gives us a good model for approaching the maladies and complications which we find ourselves struggling with: our troubles are our blessings, in that they give us a focus of attention, a doorway through which to explore what it really means to be a human being, alive on this amazing planet, conscious of ourselves and wondering what our purpose might be. Perhaps our purpose is to accept the challenge, be it failing eyesight or perfect vision which somehow does not see at all, and to follow this challenge wherever it might lead us.

Where the challenge leads you depends on your readiness to be a pioneer in the emerging field of psycho-medical healing. It is a great step in your life, to assume responsibility for your health condition, and to consciously act to improve that condition. As long as you see

[1]J. Kramer, *The Passionate Mind*, page 122 (Milbrae, Calif., 1973).

yourself as a victim, you are a victim indeed. Our perceptions of ourselves, deep down, determine for each of us what is possible and what is not impossible.

Perhaps it will take time before you really feel that you can use your consciousness to affect your eyes. I hope that you give yourself time and space and enough self-love to activate your healing mechanism.

And in this light, I should point out what most of you know already – that there are many people totally blind, who are more happy and satisfied with life than many people who can see quite clearly at the physical level but who are emotionally constricted and lacking in love and inner visions of what life is all about.

Even if you have lost most of your eyesight due to diabetes, glaucoma, or other problems, you can still use many of the exercises, meditations and programmes in this book to your advantage, because vision is more than physical, and your visual centre of your brain is also a highly active mental and spiritual centre, even when the inputs cease to flow in.

In conclusion, it appears that the most important healing is the inner healing, the emotional recovery, the expansion of consciousness beyond the old anxiety patterns and perceptual blocks. The actual physical healing is a result of the inner healing. And even if your eyesight has been too damaged physically to respond to the psycho-medical healing techniques, you can be blessed with an emotional and mental growth and evolution which keeps the inner lights burning.

As a last word on healing, I will allow Larry Dossey, one of the medical spokesmen of the emerging era of self-healing, to have the final say. In *Space, Time, and Medicine,* he writes:

> It is the sense of reverence, oneness, and unity that allows the power of healing to flower. It is the power we have lost in our age, and we may yet regain it through a new understanding of space, time, matter, and self.

With these words, we find ourselves back in Chapter 1 with the basic exercises which serve to awaken an expanded sense of space, time perception, and our own consciousness. I hope that the progression of exercises you now have available to you serves you well, continues to expand each time you do them, and brings you the healing, clarity, and insights which you desire.

So, enough said. Good luck with your eyes, with your breathing, with your evolution in general.

And in the most secular but significant meaning of the words – God bless!

John Selby

BIBLIOGRAPHY

Amigo, G., 'Pre-School Vision Study', in *Br. J. Ophtalmology*, 57/125, 1973.

Augusteyn, R.C., *The Eye*, 2 Bde., Montreal 1979.

Benson, H., *The Relaxation Response*, New York 1976.

Bronowski, A., *A Sense of the Future*, Cambridge 1977.

Brown, B., *Supermind*, New York 1980.

Carmichael, L., *Reading and Visual Fatigue*, Connecticut 1947.

Castaneda, C., *Tales of Power*, New York 1973.

Cornsweet, T.N., *Visual Perception*, London 1970.

Davson, H., Hrsg., *The Eye*, 4 Bde., London 1962.

Debos, R., *Man, Medicine and Environment*, New York 1968.

Dossey, L., *Space, Time, and Medicine*, Boulder 1977.

Duke-Elder, W.S., and L.V. Mosby, *Textbook of Ophtalmology*, 6 Bde., St. Louis 1944.

Duke-Elder, W.S., Hrsg., *System of Ophtalmology*, London 1970.

Emery, J., and L.V. Mosby, Cataract Surgery, 1980.

–, *Extra-Casular Cataract Surgery*, 1983.

Epstein, W., *Stability and Constancy in Visual Perception*, New York 1977.

Eyestrain and VDU's Symposium, The Ergonomics Society, Loughborough 1979.

Frank J., 'Mind-Body Relationships in Illness and Healing', in *Journal of the International Academy of Preventative Medicine*, Bd. 2, Nr. 3, 1975.

Gesell, A., *Vision: Its Development in Infant and Child*, New York 1949.

Girard, L., *Corneal Surgery*, St. Louis 1981.

Golas, Th., *The Lazy Man's Guide to Enlightenment*, New York 1972.

Gonzalez, C., *Strabismus & Ocular Motility*, Baltimore 1983.

Harley, R.D., und W.B. Saunders, *Pediatric Ophtalmology*, Philadelphia 1983.

Hentschel, M., 'Physiologie und psychosomatische Variablen der Myopie', unveröffentlichter Forschungsbericht,, über M. Gollub (s. S. 235) erhältlich.

Hills, B.L., 'Vision, Visibility, and Driving', in *Perception*, 9/183, 1980.

Hollwich, F., *Influence of Ocular Light Perception on Metabolism in Man and Animal*, New York 1979.

Hunain Ibn Ishaq, *The Book of the Ten Treatises on the Eye*,

Cairo 1928.

Jameson, D., *Handbook of Sensory Physiology*, Berlin 1972.

Kolers, P.A., '*Experiments* in Reading', in *Scientific American*, 227/814, 1972.

Kramer, J., *The Passionate Mind*, Milbrae, Calif., 1973.

Krieglstein, G.K., *Glaucoma Update*, New York 1983.

LeShan, L., *How to Meditate*, Boston 1974.

Liebowitz, H.W., 'Night Myopia and the Intermediate Dark Focus of Accommodation', in *J. Opt. Soc. Amer.*, 65/1121, 1975.

'Lighting for Difficult Visual Tasks', in *Human Factors*, 15/149, 1973.

Luckiesh, M., and F.K. Moss, *The Science of Seeing*, London 1980.

Lynes, J.A., *Principles of Natural Lighting*, London 1968.

Monty, R.A., *Eye Movement and Physiological Processes*, New Jersey 1970.

Mosby, L.V., *Ophtalmology*, 14 Bde., St. Louis 1961.

–, Hrsg., *Symposium on Strabismus*, New Orleans Academy of Ophtalmology, St. Louis 1971.

Moss, F.K., und M. Luckiesh, *Reading as a Visual Task*, London 1942.

Neurnberger, P., *Freedom from Stress*, Honsdale 1981.

Penfield, W., *The Mystery of the Mind*, Princeton 1975.

The Prevention of Blindness, World Health Organization, WHO Technical Reports, Nr. 519, Genf 1973.

'The Retinex Theory of Color Vision', in *Scientific American*, 237/6/108, 1977.

Rolf, I., *The Integration of Human Structures*, New York 1973.

Safir, A., *Refraction and Clinical Optics*, New York 1980.

Scholl, L., and J. Selby, *Visionetics*, New York 1975.

Schutz, J.S., *Retinal Detachment Surgery*, London 1984.

Selby, J., *Natürlich atmen*, Basel 1984.

–, *The See Clearly Book*, Santa Fe 1981 (dt. *Wieder klar sehen*).

Spencer, H., *The Visible World*, London 1968.

von Fieandt. K., *The Perceptual World*, London 1977.

von Noorden, G.K., *Theory and Management of Strabismus*, St. Louis 1980.

Waldram, J.A., *Developments in Lighting*, London 1978.

Weale, R.A., and H.K. Lewis, *The Ageing Eye*, London 1963.

Welford, A.T., *Fundamentals of Skill*, London 1968.

Wurtman, R.J., 'The Effect of Light on Man and other Mammals' in *Annual Review of Physiology*, 37/467, 1975.